LEAPFROG

A CORPORATE THRILLER BY

KIRCH P. ANDREWS

----

*Thank you for
Your support.*

[signature]

FOREWORD BY:

DR. W. GRAHAM RICHARDS, C.B.E.
CHAIRMAN OF CHEMISTRY
DIRECTOR OF THE CENTRE FOR
COMPUTATIONAL DRUG DESIGN
UNIVERSITY OF OXFORD
UNITED KINGDOM

The profits from this novel will be donated to charity.

Order additional copies at www.kirchpandrews.com

Leapfrog

First-point-five Edition

ISBN #: 1-59196-415-6

To my father, who never had the chance to read this book.

You are inspiration and to you I owe my drive.

To my mother, who wears the wings of an angel.

You are love and to you I owe my compassion.

And to Mr. Riley James, who represents all that is good.

You are my hope and future, and to you I owe all that I am.

FOREWORD BY

DR. W. GRAHAM RICHARDS, C.B.E.

Carl Djerassi, who is distinguished as an author as well as being the 'father of the pill', has highlighted the important genre of 'science in fiction' as opposed to science fiction. It is a significant category, giving the general public a sense of what science is really like. Currently a major aspect is the vital, but occasionally fraught, boundary with business. This tension introduces real moral dilemmas but also provides a fertile source for fiction.

Kirch P. Andrews has produced a perfect example. In addition to exploring the corporate-scientific hinterland, he has produced a novel of the new millennium, when the less attractive aspects of some major companies have been revealed. Much of the science discussed is real and happening today. The convergence of computer and life sciences will continue to speed the drug discovery process, help design a drug's architecture and functionality, and even personalize medicine unique to each individual.

Given the nature of the enterprise he has also chosen the most appropriate means of production and distribution for the novel. This use of computers and the Internet has a perfect resonance with his subject matter.

The work deserves a widespread readership. It will make an impact.

Dr. W. Graham Richards

PREFACE

I wrote this novel over the course of some estimated 6,000 hours and nearly eight years. The book is a corporate thriller that takes place in the cutting-edge world of drug discovery. At the time I started the book, I was pursuing an MBA in Austin, Texas and my father was suffering from a rare and aggressive form of prostate cancer. Eight months later, he was gone.

Part of my recovery was losing myself in a fast-moving business career for Dell Computer, a company on a rocket ship ride in the late 90's. I even ran my own software start-up for several years. Weeks would come and go fist fighting for further efficiency and taking at the expense of others as a way of life. At times I wondered if I even had the ability to selflessly give anything to this world.

Despite the grueling and lengthy effort, I decided to wrap up my expertise, my heart and this book and give all of the profits to charity... and get nothing in return. I don't want to pass through this earth and time without doing something, no matter how small, which leaves the world around me slightly better than before.

I hope that you, and others you know, will enjoy a copy and support me in donating the funds to the National Foundation for Cancer Research. These are the folks who can really make this world a better place. I am just a normal guy, looking into his own heart, trying to do something positive for this world. Thank you for making that dream one step closer to reality.

Kirch P. Andrews

- 1984 -

"Leave me alone!" she screamed.

Bethany Rawlins sped through the forest at a blistering pace. She'd been running at top speed for nearly twenty minutes and the long battle over the uneven forest floor was beginning to take its toll. Her breath was ragged and strained and blew from her mouth in quick blasts through cold mountain air. Swollen eyes welled with tears that streaked down the length of her pinkish cheeks and around to the sides of her neck. Her body was begging her to quit.

She glanced behind. He was still there. And gaining ground. A military shovel extended from his right hand, pumping up and down as he continued a relentless pursuit.

A rock. Branch. Another rock. Her feet sloshed through an inch-deep puddle and then disappeared again into a sea of knee-high ferns.

She leapt over a rotted log, tearing the branches from a nearby tree. A new set of lacerations appeared on her flailing arms as broken shards of wood splintered to the ground in her wake. Beth grasped at the wound, thinking instantly of her letterman's jacket left beneath the cemetery's towering pine during her frenzied escape.

"Stop running, Claire!" the young man shouted from behind.

The rage in his voice accelerated her pace. But as her legs stretched beneath the darkening canopy of Oregon firs, the tears began to fade. Her strength was tapering. It was only a matter of time before her frame would reach its limit. She had to find help.

"I'm NOT Claire," her voice cried blindly to the open forest. Things were happening fast and her vision blurred as obstacles quickly approached. A log. Rock. Branch. Another rock. "Please stop! I can't-"

Beth stumbled forward, her foot momentarily teetering on a half-stump jutting upwards from a tuft of grass. She reached a steep hill and scrambled desperately upwards.

She knew from her childhood days that somewhere over this hill was Highway 4, the main artery into Longview. For the first time, she could see the sky. It was late. Five, six o'clock maybe. Plenty of commuters traveling home from work.

Beth clawed at the earth, fighting the menacing slope. She moaned and coughed as each of her hands and feet dug deep into the soft earth, each muscle burning from exhaustion.

"Stop right there, Claire," a voice boomed from below. "Not another inch!"

He was close now and she could hear him fighting his own battle against the upward slope. Almost there. All she had to do was-

Beth's right foot slipped across the damp surface of a loose stone. Her feet clambered for traction and though she tightened her grip, her hands were slipping across the thin stock of plant holding her in place.

"NO!"

The weight of her body tore the plant from its roots and she began to slide down the muddied incline. Beth grabbed wildly at anything that would slow her descent. Her fists dug savagely into the soil, scarring the side of the hill with violent, earth-plowing strokes.

Suddenly, her body jerked to a halt. With one hand clutching the decayed branch of a fallen tree, Beth's legs swung instinctively beneath her and searched again for solid footing.

Clank.

The shovel's metal edge rang loudly as it connected with an exposed rock just beneath her foot. Beth stretched to put a second hand on the tree for more stability. He swung again, this time the blade slicing through the undersection of her sole, spinning her sideways.

Her kneecap slammed against the jagged edge of another stone, forcing an unprompted groan. The pain was sharp and she could feel the skin split open in the cool mountain air. A sudden sting gripped her stomach, her vision blurred, and the blood rushed briefly from her head.

Beth scrambled her legs, anticipating another attack but there was nothing. He'd lost his own balance and was gathering himself below. She shuffled hand over hand along the branch in search of less slippery ground. Her feet hunted for an anchor. Finally.

Beth screamed.

His fingers were locked around one of her ankles and pulling her downward. She was surprised at his strength. She could feel the bark tear at the skin beneath her palms as he clutched and pulled harder.

"You're dead, Claire!" he yelled. "You hear me? Dead!"

Beth kicked with all of her might, sending bits and pieces of earth tumbling into the man's face. But his grasp only tightened around her ankles.

She screamed louder and kicked with everything she had. Beth could feel his fingers slipping down the length of her foot. She kicked again, causing the stalker to pull the shoe from her foot and slide back down the hill. He let out a terrible growl as he threw the shoe aside and dug his own hands angrily into the damp soil to stop his descent.

Beth focused on the top of the hill, on Highway 4, and battled the incline on all fours until finally she reached a point where she could stand and locate the road.

Thank God. I-

Nothing.

Beth stared blankly over the entire valley. There were no signs of a highway cutting through the forest. No telephone poles. No buildings. No headlights. No sounds of a distant roadway.

For a brief and awkward moment she thought about Dana Vernoy, the band-camp daughter of two hippies who was covered in zits, ruined the math curve for everyone, and had two pet lizards named Elmo and Moo. Beth would need a hundred hands to count the number of times she'd thanked God, or whoever, that she was not Dana. On the contrary, Beth dedicated herself to the dance team, to everything social, and to the most controversial boys in school. This last experiment, however, was a mistake. Now all she could think about was how much she wished she were Dana Vernoy.

Splintering branches broke her empty stare. He was nearing the top. Beth bolted blindly along a high forested ridge connecting two steep hills, unaware of a thorn patch that scratched and tore through the skin on her legs. She was becoming more delirious with each passing second, struggling for each breath. As she tumbled over a fallen log, Beth felt a softball-sized rock tear past her head.

A surge of fear raced through her chest. She was starting to hyperventilate. He was going to kill her. Not kidnap. Not rape. He was going to kill her anyway he could.

As quickly as she could change direction, a second stone smashed heavily against the back of her shoulder forcing her sideways into the trunk of a large tree. Her arm fell instantly limp at her side. Beth could see him rummaging the ground for another rock as he galloped in full hunt. The pain was unbearable. She reached around her shoulder and felt a bloodied gap where the inner flesh had torn away. A flash of faintness. She had to keep moving. Beth felt the pull of her stomach, the bile rising in her throat only to fall back again.

Her legs buckled slightly as she leapt over a patch of dead branches. A third rock went flying by. She could feel herself losing hope. Her once vibrant sprint had now been reduced to a desperate canter with an injured arm held tightly against a half-bent frame.

A fourth stone slammed into the back of Beth's thigh, sending her face first into a patch of ferns. She tried to get up but her muscles were exhausted. Beth gritted her teeth and pushed, the veins in her face bulging as she stressed her body to its limit. Push. Push. Almost. Push. Almost.

She coughed, half-choked, and fell back to the ground. Her body had given all it could afford. Beth closed her eyes. For the first time she was able to relax. She was finally able to rest her body. The pain seemed to instantly disappear.

She could hear the soft crunch of pine needles as the man approached. Beth drew in her arms and legs and opened her eyes to take one last picture of the forest floor and towering pines sweeping away from her. "God's country," her father used to say. She closed her eyes. Time to sleep. Wouldn't be long now.

She could hear the man quietly circling her body until at last he had come full circle. She raised her eyelids to half-mast. Beth wanted him to see her. He did. And then he leaned over and picked up a large circular stone, hoisting it high above his head.

"Go back to hell, you stupid-"

The man's knees buckled as Beth whipped a thick wooden branch into the side of his leg. She struggled to stand as he whirled about the ground in agony. He lunged forward to grab her but she rolled quickly away.

Beth stood and limped painfully in a new direction. Although she'd managed to open a slight gap, he was almost on his feet, ready to pursue a second time. A rock. Stump. Another log. A minute later and the forest was too thick to determine how close he was to her. She'd done everything possible to escape. She desperately needed to rest.

Beth danced to avoid a grouping of trees. Suddenly her footing was lost and her body returned to the earth. She cringed in pain and clutched at her ankle, which had turned outwards to the ground. Beth quickly brought herself to her hands and knees. She looked behind but there was no one there. She waited and waited. Ten seconds. Twenty seconds. Thirty seconds.

Beth hung her head and tried to locate the pain in her ankle. The skin had ballooned up around the top part of her shoe. She shifted her weight from the swollen ankle and rose to her feet.

Beth was in shock and although she kept telling herself everything would be okay, she knew it would be dark soon and that he was still out there somewhere. Her hands trembled as she wiped the dirt and blood from her chest and face. Her shins, too, were bleeding and the criss-crossed wounds on her arms told the story of a frantic escape.

Why had she met him there? A graveyard no less. She was so stupid. Always competing for attention. And it sounded so good at the time. Melanie would never have believed she did it in a graveyard. And now look at her.

Beth froze. A noise in the distance. That sound. There was no mistaking it. An air horn from a logging truck. Highway 4. Beth was close. She was going to make it.

She moved cautiously to the edge of a steep hill, glancing down to a small ravine filled with trees. No more than fifty yards away, between the thick trunks of the Oregon woods, she could see the pale white lines defining the edge of Highway 4.

Snap.

Beth turned around and around in every direction to anticipate his approach but there was nobody there.

"Please, stop," she pleaded blindly into the woods. Her heart was racing again. Her chest tightened, her breath narrowing. "Why are you doing this to me?"

Snap.

The man approached rapidly twenty yards from her side. His soiled clothes hung loosely from his lanky frame as he gripped the shovel with two strong hands.

Beth hobbled further along the top of the ravine and, despite the agony, successfully navigated a maze of trees and rocks hooded with moss. The roadway was just below. The time was now. She turned sharply and bounded down the declining slope.

"Claire!" he yelled. "Stop, Claire!"

Beth hopped and skipped downwards, her arms flailing in every direction to slow her descent. She tried desperately to keep her injured foot from touching the ground but as her speed increased, she began to lose control.

In a matter of seconds, her body erupted through a thin fence of trees bordering the roadway's edge. Claw-like branches ripped into her arms, and then into her torso and face. Suddenly, Beth's injured foot snagged the underside of a length of barbed wire lying just above ground. Her arms shot instinctively out before her as her palms plowed through loose cinders lining the pavement's outside edge.

Smack.

The top of Beth's skull collided with the craggy edge of mile marker thirty-two, snapping her neck forcefully backwards. For the next few seconds she lay there motionless. As a small trickle of blood ran down the side of her forehead, Beth's eyes began to blink rapidly. Small twitching motions soon followed, causing her arms and legs to move back and forth in quick, shivering movements. And then all feeling was lost. Beth was alive but unable to move. Far in the distance, at the roadway's nearest turn, she could see a small blur moving slowly towards her. Surely they'd stop to help.

The shadow of a person fell over her face as the man kneeled and smiled at his reflection in her open eyes. Beth screamed but no sound was made. She could sense one of his hands grip the back of her hair while the other clutched at her dress near the small of her back. Beth shrieked in dreadful silence but the ground beneath her surrendered frame began to move in the opposite direction, and within seconds the roadway disappeared behind a wall of thick mountain grass. Ten minutes later, the tranquil mountain air was filled with the dampened sounds of a metal blade furiously displacing shovel-full portions of the forest's soil.

With two walls of earth rising slightly from either side, Beth looked between the treetops at a passing cloud. She thought again of Dana Vernoy. And then, little by little, the world went dark.

DESTRUCTION
- 1997 -

CHAPTER ONE

The sun shone brightly overhead on a glorious October morning. After five days of rain, the Portland clouds had finally disappeared and the dazzling golden sun came barreling through.

Dr. John Hawthorn approached the security gate at the rear hospital entrance reserved for doctors and professional staff. Although driving the same beat up Nissan Stanza his parents had bought him after high school, Hawthorn felt as if he were parading in a Rolls Royce. He was almost finished with his last year of residency at the Center for Medical Excellence and was practically assured a permanent position.

Hawthorn reached forward and bent the rear-view mirror to a more agreeable angle. He grinned widely, inspected his teeth, and then moved an impossible tuft of chocolate brown hair to its proper location. He tilted his chin high and examined the morning's shave. Everything looked in order.

Hawthorn glanced toward the building's front gates where two young interns framed a massive granite sign marking the main entrance. They looked nervous, hands lodged deep in white overcoats, bright blue intern badges proclaiming their ignorance. Second year researchers, no doubt. The lifeless shade of their skin gave them away.

Hawthorn looked again into the mirror and smiled. He'd been there. And everyone had a story to tell. Regardless of their social skills, he appreciated their fervor for attending what was known as the 'Top Gun' academy for the most outstanding young physicians and researchers on the planet. With a mission to supply the most gifted young minds with capital and expertise, the CME was heads and shoulders above any private or public institution in the world. The Center was staffed with the best in the business who'd guide and offer input to each young physician and researcher on a daily basis. Natural selection was alive and well here, though, Hawthorn thought. You were either part of the steamroller or part of the pavement and the CME didn't care which. 'Push the envelope or Pack your bags' was on the T-shirt at orientation.

Hawthorn had known, of course, that the odds of gaining admission to the CME once a person had finished medical school were only one in three thousand. There were no applications; only private references and outstanding achievements would gain the Center's attention.

Hawthorn draped his left arm across the steering wheel and then reached across the center console to grab his badge from the top of several Journal articles he'd read the night before.

He certainly wasn't the smartest resident but he was fiercely dedicated, studying twice as hard to compete with brains twice his capacity. He was determined as hell, or at least he liked to think so. He wanted to be the best. He'd learned long ago from his parents the value of hard work and perseverance. His father's hands, as did his grandfather's, cultivated the rich south Texas soil near Orange Grove, each year raising crops of cotton and corn to feed people they would never know. And each year was spent borrowing from the local bank in hopes that Mother Nature would provide the land enough nourishment to put food on the table.

"You pick your share, boy?" his father would ask, holding out a lantern and gunnysack.

"It's late, daddy. Football went till dark. Can I get up early?"

"Everyone's got to earn their right. Now take these, pick your share, and then get on them books. The only way you gonna get out of this mess."

The truth was, it may not have mattered what his father said. Hawthorn didn't have a choice and he knew it. He *had* to break free from the financial uncertainty of a farmer's life. He *had* to pursue a career that would one day liberate himself and his family from generations of toil and uncertainty. That was true, but he also knew of a darker balance to this humility. As time went on, he met those who had never known difficulty and he became somewhat ashamed of his background, afraid of it. Of course he was committed to excellence in his profession and to the love of his family. But what drove Dr. John Hawthorn was pure fear, and he knew it. Fear that he may not deliver. Fear that he may not be the one. Fear that he may end up like-

Hawthorn pulled along side a small guard station and rolled to a halt. He lowered his window, the manual crankshaft sticking in short jerks. A long-faced elderly man in a blue uniform leaned out of the sliding glass door. Hawthorn reached behind the passenger seat and withdrew a paperback book.

"Morning," the guard said cheerfully.

"Morning, Howard." Hawthorn held out the book and his badge. "Great story."

Howard smiled, admiring the book with his own two hands. "Vonnegut's a champ, ain't he?"

Despite the simplicity of his current occupation, Howard was an educated man and a long time chemical engineer for Dupont. He moved to Portland when his son was stricken with a rare nerve disease. His boy, of course, was brought immediately to the CME with a young Hawthorn as one of the attending physicians.

The young man had fought through a rare form of Lou Gehrig's for many months but improved rapidly with each passing day. Every night Howard would sit in the same chair. Hours at a time. He'd hold his son's head tenderly in his lap, telling him that he would soon be able to leave. Hawthorn spent many nights sitting by his side and only after the nurses urged them to go home would Howard take a small break.

Unfortunately, on the eve his son was to leave the Center, inoperable hemorrhages developed around the base of the brain. After his son passed away, Hawthorn talked Howard into staying in the area and working part-time for the Center.

"I knew you'd like it," he said, thumbing through its pages. "Couldn't put it down, could you?"

Hawthorn nodded.

"I've got more, you know. Vonnegut and I are like this," he said, intertwining two of his bony fingers. "I'll lend you another if you'd like."

"I would, although it may be a couple of weeks. Some of us can't retire just yet."

"Well, you're just a baby. Work hard play hard."

Hawthorn gave him a quick wave as he raised the window. After a bit of squealing, the gears grinded out a loud metallic sound and the car rolled slowly forward. Hawthorn looked nervously through his soiled windows to make sure no one had noticed. A new vehicle was rapidly moving up the list.

For the next few moments, Hawthorn searched for the nearest parking spot. For most, this process was considered tedious and burdensome but for Hawthorn it was like shopping with a fat wallet. He gazed carefully over each of the head physicians' cars. Chief of Surgery... Mercedes convertible... about ninety thousand... old man's car. Head of Neurological Research... Porsche 911... seventy-five grand... fun but small. Chief Executive Officer... brown Volvo station wagon... who gives a crap... what kind of an idiot would drive-

Hawthorn slammed on the brakes and the car lunged forward. Through the windshield he could see Dr. Williams glaring down on him with two hands planted angrily on the hood of the car.

"What in God's name are you doing?" Williams barked, rounding the automobile. His bushy eyebrows pinched forward, the deep wrinkles across his forehead creased with agitation.

Dr. Allen Williams had been with the Center for nearly thirty-five years and was highly praised as *the* major contributor to the hospital's success. His own brilliance as a practicing neurologist had twelve years passed, his new source of inspiration found in maintaining the world-renowned status of the medical institution he'd worked so hard to develop. Although he'd enjoyed the financial rewards of his labors for many years, the CME grapevine hinted that he was inches from personal bankruptcy. Risky investments and a brutal ex-wife, Hawthorn heard. Cost him millions.

Even worse, it was also rumored he was due to retire in less than a year and had little money with which to do so. Hawthorn surmised that Williams could have easily left the company to take a lucrative position with several private firms years ago, but the Center was his child and he had already signed his last five-year contract extension to carry him to retirement at the end of the year. Besides, no company would be willing to hire him at such an age given the benefits and salary he would need to command. The real problem was that Williams was a born general. He loved to run his center and he ran it like he was on the front lines of war.

"Dr. Williams, hello," Hawthorn fumbled. "I didn't see you crossing. I'm-"

"You're what? Driving like an idiot? Like an impatient child?"

Williams was also directly responsible for all of the Center's administrative duties, which included monitoring the progress of the various resident doctors. Hawthorn knew that Williams could make or break a young doctor's career, and although he was considered terribly old-fashioned and consistently rude, his unyielding power and influence were never in question.

"I'm sorry, Dr. Williams. I didn't see you-"

"Slow down," he interrupted. "Jesus H- I don't know why you kids are always in such a hurry. What's the rush?"

"I just didn't see-"

"Be-more-careful. You could hurt someone. My God. If you still want to park back here, son, you'll learn to be more cautious. I can take the privilege away as quickly as you received it. You understand me?" He stared Hawthorn down and then pushed himself away from the car, walking quickly towards the hospital entrance.

Hawthorn followed him in his side mirror for a while and, when he felt Williams was far enough away, pulled cautiously forward to search out a safer parking spot. He decided to try to forget this little episode. Hawthorn had a busy day in front of him and couldn't afford to be bothered with insignificant events. He was a doctor and he had lives to save.

*　　*　　*　　*　　*　　*　　*　　*

Hawthorn quietly washed his hands in the prep room before entering what he considered to be the worst of all possible situations. A one-way email from CME administration earlier in the day had requested his attendance at a routine autopsy. Although he hated to attend these grisly examinations, he realized they were part of his ongoing education and understood their importance to his career. Not until he had arrived did he realize the full implications of this 'routine' exploration.

Hawthorn turned off the water and grabbed a white towel that dangled from a metal rung on the wall. No words had been spoken in the small room for the past ten minutes as each junior physician pondered the inexplicable loss of human life under a fellow staff member's care.

"You ready for this?" he asked, tossing the towel into an empty laundry bin. Hawthorn was speaking to a colleague and friend, Dr. Mason Shane, also in his last year of residency. Actually, he was much more than a colleague. Mason was like a brother. Hawthorn would do just about anything for him. There was a time in Hawthorn's past, while attending Stanford's School of Medicine, when he'd been exposed to a deadly amount of freon from a broken refrigerator valve in his home. Hawthorn's lack of physical damage was due in large part to the medical actions performed by his roommate at the time, Mason Shane. Without Mason's quick work, Hawthorn would not be around today.

"It was no big deal, Hawthorn," Mason said. "I'm glad I was there."

The truth was, no one had Hawthorn's respect like Mason. Although his unorthodox philosophies of medicine at times strayed far from the traditional, Mason was regarded as one of the most brilliant physicians ever to grace the CME. His intelligence originated not from laborious academic work, but from natural understanding. His mind contained a natural filter for irrelevance and he questioned everything sacred to the medical field. To him nothing was a given.

"Mason, I asked you if you were ready for this."

"What do you think?" Mason snapped.

"When did you find out?" Hawthorn sat slowly on a thin wooden bench in front of a row of lockers as Mason glared sternly at a blank wall.

"Seven."

"Anything you want to tell me before we get in there?"

"What do you think this is, John? You think I got some secret to hide here? Give me a break. Christ."

"Mason, relax. I'm just trying to help."

"You think I'm waiting to tell you why this patient is dead? Is that it? You think I know?"

"Of course not."

"I have no idea. All right? I mean I have no idea."

Hawthorn glanced to the far end of the small room. Crouched over a small satchel at the far end of the room was Dr. Briggs, an overbearing second year resident who was busy rummaging through the side pockets of his bag. Hawthorn considered Briggs the worst of the lot, an arrogant doctor still reveling at the fact that he had somehow made it into the halls of the CME. Regardless of his academic brilliance, however, he seemed a mindless frat boy complete with a certain fondness for the bottle. And, although he always performed his duties with precision, that fact remained an underlying source of potential harm.

"Hate to rain on your parade, there, Mason," Briggs intruded. "But people die. Hello? People frickin' die. We can't sit here and cry for every single one."

Hawthorn motioned for Briggs to quiet down. Normally Mason would have run Briggs into the ground but this time he just stood there in angry silence.

"I just want to help, Mason," Hawthorn added. "That's all."

Dr. Hank Rector cracked open the door, stuck his chubby face into the room, and took a look at his team. Rector was the Chief of Forensic Pathology, directly in charge of all autopsies performed at the CME. He'd been with the Center almost as long as Williams and was widely expected to be the next CEO, hand-picked by Williams himself. At five-foot-nine and nearly two hundred and sixty pounds he was not the pinnacle specimen of leadership, but he'd waited a lifetime behind Williams to assume the top post and, with Williams' retirement less than one year away, all Rector had to do was stay the path and the throne would be his.

"Gentlemen, are we ready?" he asked, tucking some gray hair into his cap and adjusting his wire-rim glasses on the tip of a rounded nose. The junior physicians closed their lockers and made their way through a pair of flapping silver doors that led to the stark and sterile examining room.

Powerful lights on six-foot stands focused on the cadaver of a young female laying flat between a white sheet and a shiny aluminum table. Next to the table was a double-decker metal tray full of instruments and cutting tools necessary for the delicate procedure. Like medieval weaponry, each pickup, bread knife, and electric saw was laid out in near perfect symmetry.

Rector assumed command in an elevated chair as the other physicians gathered quietly around the base of the table. All were silent, waiting to expose the cause of this young girl's death.

Seated across from Rector was the prosector, Dr. Chen Xiao. Xiao was at the Center by way of his affluent Chinese family near Beijing and was allowed to leave the country until he completed his training at the CME. His father had arranged for everything. His housing. Education. Everything. Evidently a Minister high up in the Chinese government.

Xiao, too, was brilliant, but his passion for the study of death isolated him from any social activity with doctors outside of the Center's walls. Many of the other residents referred to him as "Lucifer" since the Pathology department was located in a section of the hospital partially below ground. The only time he was seen among the living was when he would venture up to the cafeteria or when he was required to perform an autopsy.

"Good Morning, doctors," Rector said, already displaying his patented look of concern. "Thank you all for coming."

Xiao removed the sheet, exposing the pale adolescent cadaver. Her features were unmistakably attractive although her head had been cleanly shaved for the upcoming procedure. Her skin was swollen and blue and her eyelids a lifeless shade of grayish-white.

"Hopefully we'll be able to determine a conclusive cause of death. This patient died twelve hours ago."

"Was resuscitation attempted?" Briggs asked.

"Yes. Unsuccessful, obviously." Rector scanned over the notes made by the attending nurses and then sat the folder on a nearby counter. "Dr. Shane. She was your patient, correct?"

Mason cleared his throat. "Yes. Twenty-three year old female suffering from what I believe to be a unique case of Alzheimer's." His quick and unusual diagnosis surprised those around him.

"Alzheimer's? You've got to be kidding," Briggs interjected. "At her age?" He looked to Rector for support.

Mason swallowed uneasily and continued. "While the disease is extremely rare at this age, it is not unheard of."

"What were her symptoms?" asked Hawthorn.

"The nurses reported her behavior as moody and erratic."

"Typical female," Briggs joked. No one smiled.

"Was there shrinkage of the hippocampi?" Hawthorn inquired. He recalled that the hippocampus, a brain structure believed to be important for memory, shrank in size for patients afflicted with Alzheimer's disease. Although its cause was unknown, he'd read somewhere that lab technicians were able to monitor and record its measurements using an MRI with a high spatial resolution. "No. The MRI was negative. There was nothing new. I'd been tracking her measurements for months. Everything was normal. The hippocampi were absolutely normal. Aside from the usual dementia, her symptoms did not appear life-threatening."

"Except for the fact she's dead," blurted Xiao.

For the most part, the other doctors came to disregard those types of comments. Despite Xiao's propensity for untimely words, most of the other physicians took it for just that- simply a bunch of words. Everyone knew he had a way of applying insensitive humor to times of extreme caution. Then again, Xiao was excessively competitive and, given Mason's mental horsepower, it was to his advantage to denigrate anything that might display Mason's natural abilities.

Rector took a deep breath, his eyes rolling slowly across the corpse. "Anyone care to speculate on the cause of death?"

Hawthorn again took the initiative. "Alzheimer's patients frequently suffocate if they're not on a respirator."

Mason shook his head. "No, Hawthorn. Everything was tracked. Her disease had not progressed that far."

Rector sighed as he leaned over the young girl's forehead to examine her neck. "Based on her physical appearance and records, I'd have to say she would seem to have had at least another two years before any serious effects would've set in, assuming Dr. Shane is correct. It seems we have a bit of a mystery on our hands." He shook his head and stared down at her face with great uncertainty. "Dr. Xiao, please."

Xiao smiled. "My pleasure."

Hawthorn glanced towards Mason whose face seemed to have lost more color. Xiao's comments had gone right past him. He stared pensively at the young girl, inspecting her features as if his mind was recounting those last few days.

As Xiao prepared for the use of his slicing utensils, each doctor retreated a step or two and placed a clear plastic face shield over their nose, mouth, and eyes. Once the physicians were protected, an attendant stepped forward and placed the body block beneath the young girl's chest, causing her back to arch upward to better expose the chest cavity.

Xiao stood and made a Y-shaped incision with a large scalpel that began at the front of each shoulder, curved around the breasts, and met at the bottom of the young girl's breastbone. Once this was done, the cut continued to the pubic bone making a slight deviation to avoid the navel. The incision was deep, penetrating through the skin, against the rib cage, and completely dissecting the abdominal wall.

With the incision made, the next task was to peel the skin, muscle, and soft tissue from the chest wall with a smaller scalpel. Xiao steadied himself, made the appropriate cuts, and then pulled the chest flap over the patient's face exposing the neck muscles and front of the rib cage.

Hawthorn winced.

With the rib cage exposed, Xiao grabbed the bone cutter and made one cut up each side of the rib cage. He lifted the protective human shield from the rest of the skeleton and used his scalpel to cut through the last bit of soft tissue stuck to the back of the chest wall. Once removed, the young girl's lungs and pericardial sac were fully exposed.

Hawthorn closed his eyes. He'd been over this procedure many times, but the opening of pericardial sac always made him nauseous.

Xiao switched back to his scalpel, cutting through the pericardial sac and across the pulmonary artery where it exited the heart. He stuck his finger deep into the artery to detect for any clots that may have blocked the normal passage of blood. He shook his head. Xiao then sliced through the abdominal muscles that caused the stomach wall to slide off to either side. The pale shades of her inner being were now fully exposed, the entire cavity ready for a scrupulous inspection. The physicians gathered in close around the table.

"Note. The inner organs appear to be in good condition," said Xiao, his eyes dancing over the visible entrails.

Rector reached overhead and positioned a powerful light to better illuminate the area of inspection. "Is the lab report available, Dr. Shane?"

"Lab couldn't identify cause of death. I ordered an MRS late last week and the neuron count was perfect. Her brain chemistry appeared normal."

"An ample amount of NAA?" Briggs asked.

Good question, Hawthorn thought, somewhat surprised. He'd just read a journal entry the night before noting that NAA represented acetyaspartic acid, found only in neurons. In Alzheimer's, there was a profound loss of neurons.

"Nothing abnormal."

"And the blood volume?"

Mason shook his head.

Hawthorn bent down to get a better angle on the side of her lung. "It could be possible that her lungs were diseased," he said, straightening again.

Rector reached deep within the open chest and manipulated the heart. Pulling it to the side he carefully scanned the exposed lung tissue.

"Ah... her heart appears healthy. No, there's no sign of a respiratory disease. At least externally." He withdrew his hand from the cavity. "She appears to have been completely healthy."

Hawthorn's mind raced for an answer. "Was there a history of family illness?"

Mason gave no answer. He was staring vacantly at the girl's face again.

"Mason." Hawthorn repeated. Mason glanced uneasily towards him. "I asked if there was any history of family illness."

"Nothing relevant."

For the next few minutes the team of physicians performed various medical tests on the tissue and internal organs. In the end, there were no further clues. Every road was a dead end. Every effort fruitless. There were no easy answers this day.

"Shall we?" Xiao had the Stryker saw in his hand.

"Yes. Perhaps we should examine some tissue under the scope. It may be our only chance."

As Xiao delicately moved the roll of chest skin from the front of her face, the diener moved the body block from beneath the girl's chest to a position just under the back of her head. Xiao then made one continuous incision behind one ear, over the crown of the head, and behind the other ear dividing the skull cap into a front and rear flap of skin.

Using all of his might, Xiao lodged his fingers deep beneath the front flap of skin and pulled the scalp over the young girl's face. After pulling the back flap over the nape of the neck, Xiao started the Stryker saw and made a deep cut through the thickness of the skull. Once complete, he removed the calvarium and set it aside. "Note the presence of brain tissue atrophy."

Rector removed his glasses and wiped his forehead with a clean towel that lay nearby. "Go ahead and remove a sample. Perhaps the scope will reveal some clues."

Xiao carefully channeled his knife through a thin slice of tissue as Rector held out a small cassette. When finished, Xiao put the utensil in sterilizing fluid and the doctors moved to a white countertop outlining the back of the room.

Rector pulled his chair close to the counter and delicately situated the sample onto a small metal cartridge that electronically slid into place. The physicians huddled around a nearby monitor as Rector brought his eyes to the microscope's lens. His fingers jumped back and forth between the buttons.

"Ah-hah. I see the presence of neurofibrillary tangles in the tissue." He looked up at Mason. "This would support the Alzheimer's diagnosis. Excellent work, Dr. Shane."

Mason said nothing. He stared blankly at the screen that showed small, dark marks in the tissue.

"But we're still no closer to what actually killed her."

"Maybe she committed suicide," Briggs offered.

"There's no indication of that," replied Rector. "I'm sure you can count that one out."

Across the room, Xiao was replacing the back portion of the young girl's skull. "Just another of Mason's patients come to pay us a visit."

"Shut up, Xiao," snapped Hawthorn. "Do you have anything useful to say? Ever?"

This was the second of Mason's patients to mysteriously die in the last month. The patients had no similar characteristics and although the prospects of each living a full life were small, both had treatable conditions that would allow them to live for at least another two to five years. Everyone knew Mason was dedicated to pursuing neurological research, but they also were aware of his thoroughness and perfectionism when required to treat certain patients. To Hawthorn's knowledge, these two were no exception.

The first to die was a nine-year-old boy suffering from severe epilepsy. His condition seemed ordinary at the time and, once again, the autopsy revealed nothing. Hawthorn could tell that this latest patient affected Mason deeply. Her parents were deceased, her brother serving a life term for murder in the Illinois State Penitentiary, and her grandmother was not able to be there for another two weeks.

Rector turned off the microscope and raised his voice across the room. "Dr. Xiao, since you're so willing to give your opinion, how would you like to analyze what you've seen?"

"Simple, doctor. This one ran out of time." Xiao smiled to the rest of the group as he slapped the woman's chest plate back on top of the exposed area.

"Jesus," said Hawthorn under his breath. It disgusted him that the Center would allow such barbaric behavior to exist. If only Williams knew about this.

"Dr. Shane, your thoughts?"

Mason shook his head.

Rector took one last look at the monitor that broadcast the microscope's findings to the rest of the room. "All right. I see no reason to continue this investigation. Unusual, indeed. We'll list the cause as indeterminate."

"Second case this month, isn't it Mason?" Xiao announced from afar. "My, my, how time flies."

Mason broke from the group and quickly disappeared behind two metal doors.

"Thank you for the business, Mason," Xiao called out. "And by the way, congratulations on your award. What was it?" He slowly stroked his chin. "Oh yes. Extraordinary Achievement in Neurology. Yes, that was it, wasn't it?"

"Enough, Xiao," said Rector, turning off the microscope. "That concludes the session, folks. Thank you all for coming."

Hawthorn removed his latex gloves and peeled off his top-shirt as he walked slowly past the cadaver. He seethed with anger from Xiao's comments. There was no place in medicine for that kind of crap. This was a human life they were talking about. A human life whose flame had been extinguished for no apparent reason. Hawthorn re-entered the prep room hoping to talk to Mason but his locker was closed and he already gone.

CHAPTER TWO

Mason moved briskly down one of the hospital's many hallways. He'd completed his morning rounds and was on his way to the cafeteria for lunch when Hawthorn caught him from behind.

"Mason, wait." Although Hawthorn was five feet ten inches tall, Mason was six-three and Hawthorn had to move quickly to keep up. "Mind if I join you for lunch?"

Mason shook his head. Hawthorn knew he didn't want to talk.

"Mason, I know you're upset. I'm truly sorry about your patient. Xiao was way out of line."

"Xiao? I don't care about him." That was the truth. The first time Mason had met Xiao was in his first year of residency. For some reason there was a mix-up at orientation and they were paired together for a week in the same dorm room. Mason told Hawthorn how Xiao would stay up into the early morning hours reading books and journals on pathology. One night, Mason woke up thirsty and went into the kitchen only to find Xiao crouched in a fetal position, shivering on the floor. Vampire.

"Sometimes Xiao doesn't know when to keep his mouth shut."

"Sometimes? The award means a lot to him, John."

Hawthorn knew what he meant. Both Mason and Xiao were finalists for the Brighton Fellowship, an award given to the most outstanding resident doctor and researcher in the global medical community. The award was like an Oscar in its prestige, and carried with it a $200,000 a year stipend to be used on housing, research, or anything else. Mason had never given much thought to applying for the award. A panel of senior doctors who recognized his outstanding ability in neurological research sent in his application.

The importance of this award to Xiao, on the other hand, was paramount. The financial rewards were meaningless. His family could buy the institution over and over again. By winning the award, Xiao would automatically continue his practice and research in the United States. Without it, he would have to go through a set of appeals, ultimately ending in the hands of Dr. Williams himself. Always an unknown.

"Maybe you're right," Hawthorn agreed. "He's just so damn coarse." The two men split apart to avoid an on-coming stretcher. "How in the hell did you know she had Alzheimer's?"

"I'm her doctor."

"Seriously, Mason. It's impossible to confirm Alzheimer's without an autopsy first."

"She had classic signs of dementia. Rare, but they were there. The signs were definitely there."

"Signs? What signs?" Hawthorn suddenly felt nervous, the kind you feel as a child when everyone but you knows the same secret. He wondered if had missed something. Then again, Mason wasn't stupid. Whatever it was he used to arrive at his diagnosis, it was brilliant, and it separated him from the rest of the medical world.

"The signs were there. She was having trouble with words. And there were rapid mood swings."

"I just can't believe you were able to nail that from the start." Unlike Mason, Hawthorn could care less about research. His prowess was in his rapport with each patient. At times he was criticized for becoming excessively attached to them, but in his mind there was no substitute to the human side of medicine. It could never be compromised.

Just beyond the main elevator, the two physicians encountered a stretcher pulled flush against the wall. A puzzled nurse stood nearby, examining the patient's records and charts. A clear tube ran the length of a three-foot pole connecting a plastic IV bottle to the patient's arm.

"Dr. Shane, can you please look at this?" she asked.

Hawthorn waited behind while Mason examined the patient. This is what pissed him off. He was supposed to be the expert with patients, but everyone wanted Mason's input. *Everyone.*

Removing the clipboard from the side of the stretcher, Mason withdrew his pen and wrote something down on the chart. He paused, looked down at the male patient, and continued writing.

"What is it?" the nurse asked.

Mason shook his head. He appeared perturbed. "Briggs. The dosage of Lydocaine is way too high. And Williams signed off on it."

"Would you like me to tell Dr. Willi-?"

"No," said Mason. He handed the nurse the chart. "He'll be fine. I corrected the dosage. Just keep an eye on it."

"What was that all about?" Hawthorn asked, both men continuing down the hall.

"It's Williams. That idiot needs to decide if he's a doctor or a CEO."

Hawthorn concealed a thin smile. Both Mason and Williams had an ongoing feud on the fine line between patient care and medical research. Mason claimed that Dr. Williams was biased towards residents primarily interested in treating patients. Williams, on the other hand, had expressed openly several times that Mason shouldn't be there in the first place. He thought of Mason as much too eccentric for the good of the Center. Research over patient care? Not under his watch.

Nevertheless, it was without question who was in the driver's seat. Although Williams would normally have had the authority to seriously tamper with Mason's career, he'd waited too long. Mason's reputation as the most promising neurological researcher in the world had spread to practically every corner of the medical profession. Not only was his connection to the Center important for recruiting the next crop of residents and financial capital, but he was said to be working on some of the most cutting-edge explorations known to the neurological arena.

For the past three years, Mason had laboriously been developing a new technique called CoreTex. The Center's most skeptical professionals had originally dismissed Mason's research as "lofty" and "wasteful." With time, however, these predictions were proven false. Mason had discovered a revolutionary process that would allow doctors and psychoanalysts to successfully treat the memory loss of patients suffering from Amnesia, Alzheimer's and a myriad of other neurological diseases.

Hawthorn, as it turned out, had a profound interest in Mason's research as his own father suffered from the latter stages of Alzheimer's. He'd been home to visit only two months before and not until the fourth day did his own father remember his name. Hawthorn would stare into a set of vacant and lonely brown eyes for hours at a time. It broke his heart; waiting through days pocked with unpredictable highs and lows. He desperately wanted to tell his father how much he appreciated the sacrifices made. Hawthorn never knew a man could cry so much, but each trip home drove a cold blade through his heart.

Of course, Hawthorn made it a point never to mention his father's plight. With successful genetic manipulation years away, Mason's work represented the only perceivable cure for the near future. The last thing he wanted was to put pressure on Mason and interfere with neurological research that could benefit so many. Secretly, though, the Lord's guidance for Mason's work was at the top of his prayers each and every night.

Mason had explained his approach to Hawthorn on several occasions. "You see, John, it's long been believed that subconsciously suppressed memories are the root of many cerebral illnesses. Guided imagery and suggestive hypnosis are currently two of the only ways to reach these hidden memories and the procedures are commonly employed in the treatment of varying psychoneuroses."

The problem with hypnosis, Mason went on, was that people varied in their susceptibility to the process. This meant that many times certain people were difficult to de-hypnotize. Not only could these patients suffer from False Memory Syndrome, a condition in which the patient recalled a situation that never existed, but a doctor could effectively open a can of worms that was meant to stay closed.

"This technique manipulates neuronal activity by regulating the brain's electric currents as they interact with millions of nerve cells and their interconnecting fibers."

"You're coating nerve endings with a conductive element?" Hawthorn asked.

"Right. Similar to pain medication except we can now *control* the nerve endings. I'm convinced the basic seat of memory is located within this complex maze of interacting nerve cells. Around the frontal lobes. The CoreTex process will vary frequencies to manipulate the retrieval of certain memories to the conscious level without affecting others."

Hawthorn was amazed. "A map of the human mind."

"No, John. *The* map."

It had been two years since Mason's completion of the CoreTex device and every test at the FDA's Center for Devices and Radiological Health displayed perfect results. He had already submitted his NDA for the chemical that would coat the nerve endings and their interconnecting fibers.

Because this new chemical was considered a new molecular entity and required a unique component paramount to Mason's formula, the approval process was expected to slow considerably. However, with some senior influence from the CME, Mason's formula sped through the FDA's "fast track" approval process with unheard-of velocity.

According to Mason, the tests performed at the FDA's Center for Drug and Biologics Evaluation had come back with flying colors. Hawthorn could only imagine what that meant. Many of the industry's largest companies were already lining up at Mason's door with a checkbook in one hand and a pen in the other.

"The seeds of innovation come in strange packages," Mason said. "It seemed like such a joke at the time."

Nearly six years earlier, Mason had been working for a neuro-researcher named Dr. Sylvio MacMillan as a lab assistant in the biologics area of the Stanford Center for Medical Research. Evidently, MacMillan was a fifty-year-old research genius who somehow discovered a rare enzyme located in the hearts of the Conrava Goliath Zeteki, a nearly extinct species of frog found only in the innermost regions of the Amazon.

Each day after class, Mason assisted MacMillan in researching a new theory; one that speculated that memory may be the result of changes in nerve-cell proteins. Apparently these rare amphibians contained a unique enzyme in their vascular organs which, when combined with other chemical compounds, could break down RNA. RNA was a chemical considered vital to the synthesis of memory formation.

Tragically, Hawthorn remembered, MacMillan was the victim of a hit and run one night while walking home from work. It had been four years since his death and the culprit had not been caught. There had been countless investigations but never any solid conclusions.

"The worst tragedy," Mason said. "We've lost a legend."

Exactly what effects the enzyme had were not completely known until Mason isolated it in a lab. As the story went, he ran thousands of tests on everything from worms to rodents, concluding that this rare enzyme could also be used as a stimulus for memories and dreams. Mason worked for months conducting experiments on a flatworm; a cross-eyed little creature with a brain no bigger than the period at the end of a sentence. Despite its primitiveness, the flatworm was known for its amazingly persistent memory. For instance, the worm could be taught to contract when a light was flashed. If the worm was then cut in half, the head end would grow a tail and the tail end would grow a new head. Regardless, both sections would remember what the original worm had learned. Light means contract.

The true moment of discovery came after MacMillan's death. "I've isolated the enzyme, John. This is a big step. Watch."

He took the worm, so feverishly taught to contract with light, and dipped him into the RNA destroying enzyme. What he found was that the worm's memory had been wiped clean. Not only had it forgotten all that it had learned, but its behavior suggested it was acting on a different set of memories or taught skills, perhaps hidden or subconscious faculties.

For the next few months, Mason moved up the animal ladder. With injections to mice, the same result occurred. Cats, the same. Dogs. Monkeys. Mason had discovered a chemical that, when administered in small quantities, could cause a living being capable of thought, to temporarily vacate its current memory status while simultaneously surfacing other subliminal learning patterns.

In honor of his friend, he named the chemical Slyvy-M, for Sylvio MacMillan.

Further research led to the invention of the CoreTex device and the enzyme-mapping capability. By interacting different lengths and magnitudes of electric currents with this new chemical drug, Mason was, in effect, mapping the human brain for the specific locations of memories. And the treatment was twofold. The enzyme-laden drug would coat the brain's nerve endings and trigger the release of memories while the electric currents managed which ones surfaced to the conscious level, all without affecting the patient's current mental capacity. This meant that Mason's new techniques could be the most effective method ever contrived for fighting mental illness and disease related to memory.

"The truth is, John," whispered Mason. He leaned in close. "I don't really know where the end is."

"What do you mean?"

"What if-" Mason's brows arched devilishly.

"Yeah..."

"What if this is a glimpse?"

"Into?"

"The soul. Deja vu. The invisible hand."

Although the CoreTex technique had worked flawlessly with each and every test patient, Mason had mentioned to Hawthorn a quadrant of the mind that simply would not map. The 'Gray Zone', as he called it, would surface only when the subject had been given an excessive amount of the nerve-coating drug. Each time, the patient could recall in detail a situation from what Mason considered to be a previous era of time.

"Don't you get it, Hawthorn? I'm talking about interrelational, intergenerational continuity. Think of the possibilities. Unveiling the truth about reincarnation. Whether memory stays intact from lifetime to lifetime. Reconstructing memory and learning from pieces."

"Come on, Mason. What proof do you have that those patients weren't suffering from FMS? They could've easily-"

"Close your eyes," Mason interrupted.

"What?"

"Close your eyes." Hawthorn shot him a look of warning and then reluctantly closed his eyes. "Now, what do you see?"

"Nothing."

"You're not looking."

"Of course I'm looking. It's blank. My eyes are shut."

"It's not blank, Hawthorn. Don't you see blotches of black and light? Intermixing? Moving? Reshaping?"

Hawthorn's normally furrowed brow suddenly creased sharply. "Of course. They're action potentials. They're firing from photo receptors."

"Yes, Hawthorn. That's the physiological definition. I would propose, however, that they serve a much more significant meaning. Those images are the key. Each patient was able to clearly describe them. The detail was incredible – personalities, even locations."

Hawthorn's eyes were open again, perusing Mason's enthusiasm with a sense of doubt.

"That enzyme operates like a window cleaner if you will, a screen that allows the human mind to reacquaint itself with the past. This is unprecedented territory in neurological research, John. I'm going to show the world that the Conrava Goliath species holds the key to providing clarity into our past. Clarity that will ultimately unlock a fortune of understanding."

CHAPTER THREE

Williams stared coldly at the other members of the administrative board, each of who had taken their respective seats around a large oval conference table. A member of the hospital staff, informing him of a second unexpected death, had woken him up around three o'clock in the morning.

Once before Williams endured painful questioning by countless reporters, family members, and friends. Last time, the Center had protected Mason's reputation by telling the public there was no suspected wrongdoing but that there would be a full-scale investigation. Unfortunately, the first unexplained death occurred no more than three and a half weeks ago and the lab was still gathering data. This was the second time in a month that Williams was forced to call an emergency meeting to discuss the issue at hand.

"Let's get down to business here. Early this morning, around 1:30 a.m., another of Dr. Shane's patients passed away. Dr. Rector should be here any minute with the AR, but I will tell you that preliminary information taken at the scene was inconclusive as to the cause of death. This is the second time in less than a month this has happened and I, for one, am getting tired of these meetings."

"The patient's name, Dr. Williams?" asked Susan Kinney. She was a snappily dressed woman and the head of public relations for the CME.

Williams shuffled through his notes. "Floret... twenty-three year old female... Myra Floret."

"And the assisting physicians?" asked Karl Beltman. Beltman was the CME's director of security and technology. He'd been hired away from a major defense firm three years before to install a comprehensive, state-of-the-art security system for the Center. 'Help protect the center's assets,' Williams explained. An emotionless man with plastic hair and square gold glasses, Beltman monitored the grounds, guards, and gates from a huge control panel in the middle of the CME.

"There were no assisting physicians," Williams answered. "Dr. Shane was alone. Do we have a security report available?"

"Yes. Everything appears normal," Beltman answered. The arms of his stale blue suit creased slightly as he gathered in a computer printout held between two pale hands. "No UE's on the third floor. Flow levels of equipment normal. Uniforms accounted for. Cameras and mikes clear. Everything normal."

"Fine," Williams snapped, his fingers tightly wrapped around a cup of coffee. "A police report has been filed which means we have twenty-four hours before the public eye comes zooming in on us. Susan, I asked a personal friend at the station to delay as long as possible until we can put together some kind of statement. I'm sure the newspapers are all over them."

When the first patient had passed away, the hospital put off dealing with the police until the last minute. It was not uncommon for a patient to die with no explainable cause. Because this girl was the second in such a short period of time, Williams decided it would be in the Center's best interest to proactively file a public report. Anything to protect the Center's reputation.

"And if they ask whether or not the investigation will be criminal?" Susan asked.

Williams looked around the room. This was a difficult question. The previous death showed no sign of any physical tampering but there was also no biological explanation. Surely, a second death would bring the highly praised center under intense public scrutiny. "As long as there is a definite biological explanation for this young girl's death, I see no reason to pursue anyone."

The main door swung open and Dr. Rector quickly found his seat. His pudgy face paled with uncertainty.

"You have the results?" Williams asked.

Rector nodded. "Examination was held this morning and- and everything's negative. We can't find a thing."

"Susan, scratch that remark. This is the second time in less than a month. We cannot ignore it. You can tell the press there will be an investigation into all possible scenarios."

"And what about Dr. Shane, Allen? Is he not our best player? Our prized possession?" This was Dr. Roman Clark, the long time chairman of the board and founder of the CME. He had personally recruited Williams long ago to help build the Center to its present state. Clark was older, in his late seventies, and had once served as Commissioner of the FDA before founding the CME. Although he spent less and less time at the hospital, he occasionally dropped in from his house in the hills to sit in on a meeting. This particular problem seemed to capture his undivided attention. The reputation of his center was at stake.

Williams looked nervously around the room before addressing Clark's question. "Roman, certainly the hospital can no longer ignore the single common thread that links these two pointless deaths. Now, I'm not saying that Dr. Shane is guilty of any wrongdoing, but I do think in order to protect the institution from any unnecessary legal liability we should remove him from his privileges."

"With all due respect, Dr. Williams, that will not be necessary." Dr. Sarah Brenner removed her reading glasses, pushed back her chair, and rose to her feet. She was a middle-aged, well-established physician with sandy blonde hair and an aggressive southern tongue. "There is absolutely no reason for Dr. Shane to be suspended or reprimanded in any capacity. As head of the investigation committee, I can assure you all that, to this point, there is not the slightest bit of evidence indicating Dr. Shane is involved in any wrongdoing."

Williams placed his finger solidly on the table and rose from his seat. "Dr. Brenner, with all due respect to you, my dear, two of his patients are gone and we, the hospital, have no alternative evidence except that Dr. Shane was their attending physician. Now please take your seat."

"I disagree, Dr. Williams," Brenner replied a second time. She did not appreciate the 'my dear' comment. "Given the number of patients Dr. Shane has seen over the last two months, two deaths are not out of the ordinary."

"Are they above the mean?" Clark asked. Williams slowly returned to his seat.

"I suppose taken on a yearly basis they would be, but I think it premature to punish a young doctor for deaths that may have nothing to do with his level of expertise. We can't accuse one of the world's top talents of murder simply because our forensic team can't find a reasonable explanation for two deaths."

Rector shrugged his shoulders and rolled his eyes.

"If I may, Dr. Williams," said Dan Schwarz, the Center's lead attorney. "I think Dr. Brenner has a valid point. For the administration to dismiss Dr. Shane without substantial evidence supporting "good cause" would be a contract breach of his employment agreement. I suggest that no drastic steps be taken until the investigative committee has completed their work. To do otherwise would be premature from a legal standpoint and may open the Center to wrongful discharge and a whirlwind of controversy."

Williams did not like that answer. "I understand that, Dan, but the hospital must take some measure. Sooner or later, the public will get wind of this and all hell will break loose."

"Can we meet with Dr. Shane and ask for his cooperation?" chimed Schwarz, the Center's general counsel. "Perhaps he would agree to temporarily restrict his activities to research."

"No, no, no. I don't think that's a good idea," snapped Williams. "Either he's in or he's out. The public will eat us alive if they know a physician is under investigation for two deaths but still allowed to move freely upon the premises."

"Then why don't we just suspend him with pay?"

"He'll never go for that," said Brenner. "He doesn't care about the money. He's interested in his research. He's told us that a million times. I move we table the discussion of Dr. Shane's future until my investigation committee has had time to draw its final conclusions."

"And if another patient dies?" Williams asked.

The room fell quiet. Williams' steel-blue eyes connected with each one of them. They were all cowards as far as he was concerned. Of course Mason was dedicated to his field. Of course he preferred research over patient care. It was ridiculous to give him the benefit of the doubt with two patients gone and who knew how many more were to come.

"I'll have the committee's findings to the board as soon as possible," Brenner answered. "Until then, there is no evidence against Dr. Shane and we must give him the benefit of the doubt until scientific conclusions can be drawn."

"I agree," said Clark. He stood slowly with the help of a cane. "To suspend him prematurely could have detrimental ramifications on his career and on the reputation of this institution."

"And if another patient dies?" Williams repeated. "Who will accept responsibility?" The silence was making him sick.

"If there is no evidence against Dr. Shane, the Center will be free of any negligent position," said Schwarz.

Williams shook his head, visibly disappointed by the situation. He was the one who would have to face those annoying reporters, each of them asking who was at fault and him standing there again without an answer. "Is everyone in agreement here?"

The group members nodded.

"All right, then," he said, displeased. "We'll proceed the same way as the last time. Susan, has your office been contacted yet?"

"Yes."

"How many?"

"Two so far."

"Who?"

"Channel four and nine."

"Who from channel four?"

"Katie Burns."

Williams shook his head again. "I'll take care of her."

Williams hated Katie Burns. She'd once interviewed him to discuss some of the research done at the Center on mice. When the show was aired it made the CME look like the hot spot in North America for animal cruelty. Everything about the show was misleading. Two weeks later she called and apologized but by then she had received her huge ratings and several animal rights groups had made the hospital's front lawn their new gymnasium.

"No one speaks to the press unless it's through Susan's office or authorized by me. God help us for this decision, folks. I hope we're right. I will notify you all of any new developments through your secure accounts. And

Dr. Brenner," he added directly, "I will personally monitor your committee's progress."

Brenner said nothing as she gathered her materials from the top of the table. Only Dr. Williams remained, staring hopelessly into his notes and then to the ceiling. He knew what was coming and it was never an easy thing to do.

CHAPTER FOUR

Two hours later, Williams was sitting nervously at the edge of an executive leather chair behind an eight-foot mahogany desk. His office was overpoweringly conservative. Facing the front of his desk were two high-backed Victorian chairs located on either side of a polished cherry table. A waist-high cabinet ran the length of two sidewalls and was spotless with the exception of a family photo or two. Handcrafted, brass lamps. Persian rug. Even a late 1800 French-style armoire emblazoned with his initials held anchor to resist the passage of time.

Williams stared pensively at a printout of Mason's personnel file. Located in these documents was an array of private information ranging from Mason's physical history to an extensive psychographic profile. His eyes scanned meticulously over each line item through a pair of half-frame glasses resting on the edge of his pointy nose. The events regarding Mason's patients over the last three weeks were taking their toll on Williams' ability to endure the idiocy of those around him. As far as he was concerned there was absolutely no excuse for not taking swift and decisive action. Two deaths? My God, what in the hell were they waiting for?

Finally he reached it, a series of historical psychological tests and evaluations. He looked quickly over the dates until he'd located the right one. Williams sighed. It was all right there in black and white. He pushed the report halfway across his desk, leaned back, and stared blankly up at the ceiling. He'd sworn to himself many times never to use that information. Making it public would no doubt ruin Mason's career and certainly taint the Center's reputation. To use it against an employee for any reason contradicted the very cornerstone on which his great institution was based.

He pulled the report back across the desktop and re-read the damaging information. Given the recent events, however, the question was not if to use it but when. After all, the future of the entire center was at stake. It was *his* back that was against the wall. It was *his* ass on the line here. After reaching the last page, he gathered the stack of papers, organized them into a neat pile, and slipped them inside one of the desk drawers.

Williams picked up the phone and dialed a number in Colorado. He tapped his pen against a stone paper holder while he waited for the call to go through.

The line was busy.

He hung up and gazed vacantly across the room. What a mess. Williams could feel the stress biting in his stomach.

A green light flashed on his monitor and Williams leaned forward to take hold of the keyboard. He loved technology for the power it gave him.

"Security, control, and total information awareness, Karl," Williams said in their first meeting. "Don't worry about the money. I want lockdown here."

And together they invested significant CME dollars towards protecting the data and research beneath his wing. He went as far as making each physician sign a non-compete, non-disclosure agreement with a $500,000 dollar penalty which meant that any research being done at the CME was going to stay there for quite some time.

As far as he was concerned, the only way to achieve complete security was through absolute control. Each physician and researcher was forced to keep his or her records, measurements, and transcripts on a central database that was hand-designed by Beltman for maximum security. Although each doctor could easily access his or her own work at anytime, only Williams could access everything. This would prevent a disgruntled researcher from leaving with someone else's idea. It allowed Williams to effectively "lock out" anyone from their own research should they choose to leave the CME. It also gave Williams total visibility into everything that went on.

A shiny gloss covered his eyes as the screen lit up and named its parameters. Ten seconds later, the screen read:

-PASSWORD?

His fingers danced speedily over the keys.

-VERIFICATION?

He typed it again.

-STAND BY FOR PHYSICAL IDENTIFICATION...

The cursor blinked rapidly and then disappeared into a sea of black. Within seconds the computer screen split into two separate halves. The section on the left had a two-dimensional chart with a zigzag line connecting the tops of several colorful bars. Plotted beneath were the words "Dr. Allen Williams." The right half of the screen remained blank with the exception of four bold words across the top:

-VERNACULAR RECOGNITION SEQUENCE READY...

Williams reached for a long pen-like lever at the side of his computer, pulling it downwards like a gambler drawing the lever on a slot machine. He spoke slowly and deliberately into the tip.

"Dr. Allen Williams."

The right half of the screen changed from black to a chart identical to the left side. Moments later the computer moved the graph on the right to a position directly on top of the left half to show a perfect match. The system beeped as the screen flashed again to darkness.

-GOOD AFTERNOON DR. WILLIAMS...

The screen erupted into several brilliant colors and then arrived at the intended destination. Peering anxiously at the screen through his rectangular glasses, Williams' fingers continued to pound the keys.

-C>: VIDEOTRANSIT

This was the command to enter a secure, video-conferencing communication system. This software, although compatible with any other video conferencing system, was specifically designed for Dr. Williams' and the Center's use. Beltman developed it with features that would ensure the secrecy and security of the CME's local area network when connecting with sister nodes across the globe.

-DR. ALLEN WILLIAMS CONFIRMED... PROCEED...

The screen changed instantly to a computerized version of a Rolodex. He carefully positioned the cursor above the advance button and slowly rolled through each phone number. There it was. Geniomics, Inc. He touched the Internet address and the computer automatically dialed the number.

-LINK ESTABLISHED... transmitting sequence

Williams tightened his tie and adjusted a small camera that rested on the top part of his monitor. After patting down the side of his thinning hair, he tapped a button that read "PHANTOM." This feature allowed Williams to contact select Internet locations outside of the Center without an official record of a communications transfer. In effect, it scrambled the transmission so that the phone lines, routers, switches, ISP and the local server could not register an outgoing signal. It also enacted a compression and triple-DES encryption sequence that would further scramble the transmission in the event of a mid-line breach.

A couple of three-dimensional icons appeared at the top half of the screen. One was an external picture of the

CME and the other a photographic rendering of the Geniomics headquarters in Seattle. Connecting them was a rotating disk that appeared to spin in mid-air and travel along an arc between the two buildings. Depending on who was transmitting the signal the disk would switch directions.

A small box suddenly appeared in the lower quadrant of the screen. Centered in its frame was a man with slicked black hair, thin, angular eyebrows, and a sharp, angled nose. He wore an expensive suit and was chewing ice.

"Hello, Allen," said the man, his voice instantly condescending. The other man was Randy Edmonds, the aggressive thirty-eight year old CEO of Geniomics, Inc. Although he had originally started his corporate career with a high-tech telecommunications firm just outside of San Jose, his chemical engineering background and entrepreneurial spirit soon took over. At age twenty-three, Edmonds founded the Seattle-based, Geniomics Incorporated with fifteen thousand dollars. The pharmaceutical giant's market value was currently set at well over $80 billion. More impressive was the fact that in two short weeks they would announce to the world, the first ever cure for the common cold.

A massive publicity campaign had already begun. Television. Talk shows. Tabloids. Newspapers. Radio. Everywhere one looked, Geniomics' name was in the spotlight. Their new drug was labeled everything from "the most significant discovery of the 21st century" to "a sign of the second coming of Jesus Christ." The only remaining barrier was to finalize some minor, ancillary tests before the FDA's approval hearing in eight short days.

Williams adjusted the VRS mike at the side of his monitor to better capture his voice. "Randy, just calling to see how things are going."

Edmonds' image jerked slightly as Williams' system decoded each frame and data signal. "No glitches so far. Things are progressing as planned."

"Is the money in place?"

"Yes, Allen. Again. He better take it this time." Williams felt suddenly uneasy. "He will. This is more than he's ever seen. I don't anticipate any problems."

"Good, though I'm not terribly impressed with your skills to anticipate." Edmonds tapped his own finger against his desktop camera, the image filling Williams' screen. "You provide me with solutions, you got that? Money will be available by five o'clock today. He better take it, Allen."

Williams' smiled nervously. "I'm sure he'll be interested. This is an incredible opportunity for him."

"Damn right it is."

"Another patient died today."

Edmonds' eyes brightened perceptibly. "Good for me."

"Yes. I suppose that is good for you." Williams unlocked a drawer and took out a copy of Geniomics' financial reports. He set the document beneath the desk lamp and thumbed slowly through each page. "And the approval?"

Edmonds' winced. "That's another story. Those idiots in DC scrutinize every goddamn detail. But I've got a couple of friends who owe me. Things should be taken care of."

"And the testing is still on schedule?"

"We'll see."

Williams frowned. "What's the timeline we're looking at here?"

"Tests will be ready. That is not your concern, Allen. Is there a problem?" Edmonds asked.

"Of course not. But Shane's memo will specifically draw attention to those tests. We need to make that deadline. We need to pass and be ready to move."

"Who the hell do you think you're talking to, here?" Edmonds asked, his face suddenly tense. "Don't you think I know that? One thing at a time. You take out the risks on your end. This will be the biggest damn thing of the modern era."

"I hope so."

"Just do your part, Allen."

Before he could reply, Edmonds had terminated the link-up. Williams exited the system and stared irritably across the room. He felt unsure. Unsatisfied. He picked up the phone and re-dialed the Denver number. It was still busy. He hung up and then leaned back into his chair, closing his eyes and placing his hands on his head. He wasn't happy with what Edmonds had told him. Things were getting messy and he needed help in cleaning them up.

Williams rolled back through his electronic Rolodex and quickly jotted down a new phone number. A local number. He turned off the computer and punched his intercom button to get an outside line.

"Good afternoon, KVTL-Channel Four, can I help you?" said a friendly male voice.

"Yes," answered Williams, his thin hands gripping the armrests of his chair. "Get me Katie Burns. I have some information I know only she can appreciate."

CHAPTER FIVE

With the day's end near, the hospital cafeteria filled with the usual mix of visitors and late afternoon staff. Occasionally a group of scrub-wearing personnel would enter, chitchatting over the latest surgical success. Everywhere there were family members, some debating whether to let grandma go and others anticipating the return of their youngest child. Many expressed uncertainty while others elation that their loved ones would soon join them again in the sanctity of their own homes. It was a circus of emotion.

"Mason, you really should eat something," said Hawthorn, scraping the last bits of meat from a chicken breast with his fork.

Mason said nothing. He was staring intently through the window at the Center's main parking lot.

"So... what's the latest?"

"On?"

"The project. It's probably been two weeks since we last spoke."

"There's not much to tell."

"Nothing?"

"Passed CDER."

"You serious? That's great."

"I guess."

"Mason, look at me." Mason reluctantly turned his head. "Clinicals are done, Mason. You're there. You've made it to '3-B'. The feds go thumbs up here in a couple days and you're- Who's contacted you? Pfizer yet?"

Mason nodded his head.

"And the terms?" Hawthorn asked with an envious grin. He could only dream of being in Mason's shoes.

"We haven't got that far."

"Jesus. I'm sure it'll be huge." A busboy arrived and removed some empty glasses. "When's the séance?"

"It's an approval hearing, John. On the 24th."

Hawthorn's boyish grin rapidly disappeared. Mason hadn't caught the joke. Hawthorn knew the FDA's approval hearing for Mason's memory-coating drug was just around the corner. Each new chemical to be used for pharmaceutical purposes in the marketplace was required to pass several tests before it could be sold to the general public and Mason's drug had blazed through the FDA's traditional sequence with unthinkable speed.

One reason for the expeditious review was probably the magnitude of Mason's innovation. Typically a pharmaceutical firm would have an extremely difficult time acquiring any rights to an animal on the global endangered species list. According to Mason, these frogs were federally protected from illegitimate use by US corporations through the International Conservation Consortium - an international convention, signed by all countries to protect and regulate the trade of endangered species.

A further complication was that, in order to extract the appropriate enzyme for this new use, the animal had to be destroyed. Despite the odds, however, it seemed as if the potential of Mason's research to cure mental disease was well worth the cost and this groundbreaking research was expected to give him exclusive access to the limited medical use of the Conrava Goliath species.

Hawthorn pushed his plate away and rocked backwards in his chair. "I just want you to know that I think what you've done is incredible. I'm proud of you."

Mason had hardly heard the comment.

"Mason."

"What?" He was looking across the room at a young girl slumped over a tray of uneaten food. She wore a patch over one eye and appeared disheartened. Alone.

"Are you okay?" Still no answer. Hawthorn glanced at the girl and then back to Mason. "Are you nervous about tonight?"

"Haven't given it much thought. You going?"

"Are you serious? Jesus, I wouldn't miss it for the world. There is no recognition higher than this, Mason."

"It's just an award, John. There are more important things."

"Enjoy it. Enjoy the damn award. Hell, I wish I had it."

Mason placed his cup of coffee on the table and leaned in close, lowering his voice. His face darkened perceptibly. "I don't know, Hawthorn. I must have missed something. That girl should never have died."

"Come on, Mason. That was tough. Even Rector didn't have a clue. What else could you have done, huh?"

"Saved her."

"How? There was no way- there *is* no way to tell. How, Mason? What else?" Mason gripped the seat of his chair and tottered slowly back and forth. "Nothing. There was absolutely nothing you could have done."

"Maybe I'm not the flawless-"

"Don't even say it. You're the best there is and you know it."

"I'm worried, John. I'm worried I missed something. Remember back in med school when I had those headaches?"

Hawthorn nodded.

Mason shifted uncomfortably in his chair. He hesitated and then spoke in a tight, troubled voice. "I never told you the entire story. They were after blackout periods. Hours at a time. I had no idea where I was or what I had done. For hours, John. No recollection whatsoever."

"But you saw specialists."

"Yeah, but they couldn't tell me anything. One thought blood pressure. Another epilepsy. They even looked for tumors. No one knew. Just the other day, I woke up in the hallway. No idea how I got there. And dreams. The dreams are so intense. But I can't remember any of them. No details. Just blurs, you know? Visions. And now, this girl. A second time? I honestly can't remember anything."

"I understand, but trust me. There was nothing you could have done on this one. Okay?" Mason was again staring at the girl with the patched eye. "Okay? Everything will be fine."

Mason looked back across the table with great uncertainty.

Hawthorn grabbed his tray of food and dumped it into a large plastic bin next to the table. Mason remained quietly in his chair, gazing doubtfully through the window.

"Don't worry, Mason. Everything'll be fine. We'll get that head of yours checked tomorrow sometime. But really. There's nothing else you could have done. I'll see you later tonight."

Mason nodded and faked a smile.

As Hawthorn left Mason sitting there alone, his instincts told him that the cause of this behavior went far beyond the morning's autopsy. He'd never seen Mason this rattled before. A couple of blackouts and an inexplicable death could surely cause some stress but there was more to it than that. Hawthorn could feel it.

CHAPTER SIX

Hawthorn straightened his bow tie and entered the massive CME auditorium, navigating his way through nearly four hundred and fifty doctors, family members, and friends now gathered for the evening's awards ceremony. For the first year in the history of the CME, the prestigious center would host the ceremony for the coveted Brighton Fellowship. For one night, the entire medical field would focus on Portland, Oregon and the Center for Medical Excellence.

Hawthorn found his seat ten rows from the front and watched an elegant crowd mix and mingle as they waited with great anticipation. While some doctors shook hands and flashed transparent grins to their colleagues, their wives glared at each other's formal gowns with a sneering eye. Each man was dressed in full tuxedo and each lady in their finest evening gown. It was clearly a time to see and be seen.

Hawthorn waved to a nearby colleague.

The rest of the crowd, he knew, was there for one reason. Mason was the first person west of the Mississippi to win the Brighton Fellowship since the inception of the award in 1920. Each year the awards committee had given it to a researcher at Harvard or another eastern institution and had ignored the emerging Center in the Pacific Northwest. This time was different.

A large blue curtain, emblazoned with the silver chevron signifying the excellence for which the institution was globally renowned, served as the backdrop for the ceremony. Five speakers, including Dr. Williams, sat on each side of an oversized podium that divided the stage in two. Each wore a ritualistic black gown with a symbolic hood draped neatly over their back. Mason seated himself in the front row next to the other award finalists which included Dr. Kenneth Howard, a third year resident from Harvard specializing in neurosurgery; Dr. Jill Abrhams, a radiologist from Northwestern; and Dr. Chen Xiao.

A tall man approached center stage, stretched his claws around the mike, and spoke. "Thank you all for coming. Please allow me to introduce Dr. Sarah Brenner, Chief of Neurological Research here at the Center for Medical Excellence and one of the world's leading experts in brain tumor research. Dr. Brenner."

In addition to her outstanding medical achievements, Brenner was a long-time friend and mentor to Mason. Hawthorn had worked with her as well and knew she'd done everything possible to recruit him upon his graduation from Stanford. She once risked an illegal recruitment trip to answer any questions and concerns he might have had. Brenner saw Mason's potential from a mile away and was determined to mold him into her protégé.

"Thank you, ladies and gentlemen. Thank you," she said, organizing her notes. "This year I have the distinct honor of presenting the coveted Brighton Fellowship. This award recognizes excellence in medical research on a global scale. It is considered the highest honor given to emerging physicians and researchers in the world."

"As a young boy, this year's recipient lived with his grandfather on the Navajo Indian reservation for nearly six years. His grandfather's knowledge of traditional Indian healing led to his current interest in modern medicine."

Hawthorn glanced at Mason who sat emotionless in the front row. The crowd quietly mumbled their surprise and interest as Brenner continued. Hawthorn, of course, was one of a handful of people who could apply any detail around Mason's past. Upon the tragic death of his parents, an eleven-year-old Mason was forced to live with his grandfather on the vast and arid Navajo reservation in the northeast corner of Arizona. Mason had plenty of stories about his grandfather but never really engaged in discussions about his parents. He carried no pictures, no mementos, nothing. Hawthorn figured it was a sore spot so he never pushed the issue. The accident must have been pretty traumatic.

Six years later, Hawthorn learned, when his grandfather passed away, Mason was sent to a boarding school back in Portland where he quickly surpassed his classmates. The teachers had never seen anything like him. He could take a two hundred-page book and recite verbatim any passage from any section at any time. Mason always attributed his academic success to a superior memory, but Hawthorn knew it was more than that. Mason was truly something special.

"Pursuing this interest in healing," Brenner continued, "he graduated from Lewis and Clark University with honors in only two years and then went on to post the highest scores in the nation on his MCATs."

Xiao shuffled uncomfortably in his seat. Listening to this must have been painful. After all, his scores and accomplishments were just as impressive and Xiao came from a country where a quality education was almost impossible to acquire. Unless your father could serve up capital punishment like shrimp cocktail, of course.

"He then attended medical school at Stanford, where he graduated at the top of his class. In his last year of residency he has established himself as a highly promising talent in neurological research. Ladies and gentlemen, please join me in recognizing Dr. Mason Shane."

Brenner stepped from the podium and led the crowd in their appreciation for Mason's efforts. As a resident at UCLA, she'd been mentioned as a finalist for the award but had lost by a very slim margin. Hawthorn figured she'd anticipated this event as long as anyone and was finally able to live her dream through her young apprentice.

The crowd roared as Mason was greeted briefly by each of the distinguished guests. Two people down he met Dr. Richard Moss, the Commissioner of the FDA. Mason even shook hands with Williams who smiled cheerfully and patted him on the back.

When the crowd returned to their seats, Mason cleared his throat. The microphone gave off a short squeal. "Thank you, Dr. Brenner. And thank you to the Brighton Foundation for giving me this great honor."

"During the six years I spent with my grandfather, I learned there are many ways to heal. My grandfather was a shaman, or what you would call a medicine man. He used the knowledge of his ancestors and their belief in the spirit world to heal his people with the most primitive of means."

Hawthorn could see Xiao tilt his head with a quiet chuckle. What the hell was he laughing about? It wasn't like the Chinese were doing *in silico* research in every village.

"My ancestors believed that a person was formed by a combination of spirits found in the heart, the sky and in fire. A physical disorder was attributed to an imbalance in these spirits, and such an imbalance could often have dire consequences on the physical being."

"I believe," he continued, "that the human mind contains many secrets, and that this primitive explanation of physical disorders may be far more accurate than we know. My own research has led me to explore these questions."

"I'm sure that each of us has, at some time, been puzzled by our own actions, as if we were momentarily controlled by something other than our own conscious self. What about Deja vu? The fact that you could swear you had been somewhere even though you knew you hadn't. Or had you?"

Mason had secretly shared with Hawthorn his intentions of using the CoreTex process to possibly uncover the mystery surrounding Deja Vu. His preliminary feeling was that its source was located somewhere within the "Gray Zone" quadrant of the memory map.

"Modern medicine can no longer ignore these phenomenon. As a profession, we must be willing to challenge contemporary techniques and, at times, revisit traditional methods and ideas. There *is* more to the mind than matter. There is a connection. A power to be reckoned with. Seen. Experienced. Felt. Mathematical science is not always the answer. All too often we are trapped by what we see in books, by what we are taught in a seminar or classroom, by today's five senses. It is our responsibility, your responsibility, to unlock this hidden treasure. In the very near future, I will provide this evidence. Thank you."

The auditorium filled with a warm applause as Mason glanced uncomfortably to the others on stage. He then gave a half-wave to the crowd, lowered his head and descended to his seat.

"Mason," Hawthorn called from behind. He'd managed to fight his way through the crowd, descending a side isle to greet him.

For the next few minutes, they spoke of meeting at Dr. Brenner's for a small post-awards reception. Mason wanted to go home but eventually gave in to Hawthorn's plea. They shook hands and left the building.

"John? John." It was Dr. Williams storming Hawthorn's direction as he opened the door to his car. "Have you seen Dr. Brenner?" There was an urgent ring to his voice.

"No sir."

"If you do, tell her I need to speak with her as soon as possible. Do you understand?"

Hawthorn put his hands in his pockets. "Yes. Of course."

"Hawthorn, do-you-understand?" he barked. "I highly suggest you find her. It's very, very important."

"Yes, sir, I understand."

Hawthorn watched Williams barrel down a long row of parked cars and into the blackness of night. What was his problem? The ceremony went perfectly. Besides, Hawthorn couldn't remember the last time Williams had acknowledged his presence, regardless of the circumstances, let alone approached him for help. His only recollection of conversation with Williams was a series of weekly one-way mandates to Hawthorn's e-mail account or Hawthorn's unanticipated attempt at making him a hood ornament.

"I highly suggest you find her?"

CHAPTER SEVEN

Hawthorn's beat-up Stanza rolled carefully to a stop beneath the dull orange glow of an overhead parking lamp in the middle of the CME lot. At 9:15, the area was mostly vacant with the exception of those employees working in the emergency center and the doctors called in for the night. At Brenner's request, Hawthorn planned to stop by his office and pick up some documents regarding patients where both he and Mason had collaborated. From there he'd join them at the party.

The sliding glass door parted as Hawthorn entered a sharply decorated lobby. It was more an atrium than a greeting area, complete with modern furniture, art deco paintings, and beautiful life-size statuettes. Williams had spent a good portion of the Center's initial endowment on the appearance of the lobby. Anything to impress potential benefactors. Grab 'em and lock 'em down.

Hawthorn waved hello to Mabel, an elderly woman behind the information desk, and then waited for the elevator to take him to the fifth floor where the physician offices were located. He stared at his reflection in the bronze elevator doors. He looked tired. Sleep wouldn't come soon enough.

As the elevator came to a soft halt, Hawthorn opened his wallet, removed a shiny silver card, and slid it through a vertical slip situated next to the row of numbered buttons. A red light switched to green and Hawthorn stepped into a low-lit hallway.

The third floor was home to all CME patients. Something told Hawthorn that given the recent events, he should check on Mason's patients before attending Brenner's reception. He knew Mason was skating on thin ice and it wouldn't be long before Williams made a move.

The last thing Mason needed was another mishap. He quickly scanned the names and room numbers on his clipboard.

At this time of night, the hallways were considerably quiet since most of the patients were fast asleep. The dim overhead lights reflected a soft radiance on the tiled floor. An occasional nurse dressed in traditional white garb would emerge from one room only to dart quietly into another. Hawthorn tucked the clipboard beneath his right arm and walked unnoticed down the hall, his footsteps echoing crisply throughout the empty corridor. Within moments he was at the first room: 315.

Hawthorn leaned against the closed door to listen for voices. Satisfied, he turned the metal latch and entered the room. After making a quick read of the vital signs monitor, he retreated back into the hallway and closed the door.

The next patient was in 349. This room was located on the other side of the nurses' station at the far end of the wing. He paced quickly down the hall, careful to avoid abandoned wheelchairs and other hospital equipment left in his path.

As he rounded the corner of the main hallway, Hawthorn froze. A man dressed in a white cafeteria uniform broke from a patient's room and walked quickly towards the stairwell exit. He glanced to his clipboard. 349. At this hour only qualified nurses and physicians were allowed on the floor. This man was clearly neither.

The nearest door read 333. He moved hastily to the next. 335.

His walk soon blended to a nervous jog. 341. 343. 345. The man had come from 349. As Hawthorn quickened his pace, he briefly considered that someone could be tampering with Mason's patients. But it made no sense. Mason had no enemies and if someone did want to meddle with his career, why wouldn't they focus on his research?

At this point, it didn't matter. That man should never have had access to the third floor. The only entrance into the third floor was through the elevators with a security card. The hallway doors leading to the stairwell were "exit only" as the law required for safety reasons, so he couldn't have come up through the stairs.

Hawthorn burst into the stairwell and zipped down the stairs. His hands squeaked as he flung himself around each hairpin turn. He couldn't stop thinking of what the man may have done. The girl. The young boy a month before. Leaning over the rail he could see the man push open the door on the first floor.

"Hey!" Hawthorn yelled, descending at a rapid pace. He heard the door slam shut. A moment later, he arrived at ground level, blasting open the door. "Hey!"

The man walked calmly down the hall, doing nothing to acknowledge Hawthorn's voice.

"Hey!"

The man finally noticed Hawthorn and immediately stopped. Red stains streaked in every direction near his lap.

"Can you show me some ID, please?" Hawthorn asked, cautiously approaching. His heart was about to blow out of his chest. The man shrugged his shoulders and his eyes bounced between Hawthorn and the kitchen door behind him. "What were you doing on three?"

The intruder refused to speak. He looked at Hawthorn with nervous, bloodshot eyes.

"Answer me!"

The man flashed some sign language with his hands and then withdrew from his pocket an employee badge complete with photo and job title. He handed it to Hawthorn. Jud Parks. It looked valid. Still, Hawthorn thought, he shouldn't have been able to enter the third floor. The Center's security system required a person to have a magnetically striped card to enter so he had to have gained entrance through the elevator.

"How did you enter?" Hawthorn pointed to the ceiling and showed him three fingers, still maintain a cautious distance.

The man reached deep into his other pocket withdrawing a shiny silver security card, which read "Dannette Marco." He pointed towards the kitchen.

Dannette was the Head of Kitchen Operations for the entire center. At times she would allow one of the workers to deliver a late night meal but only with a physician's approval. Even so, this was a matter that needed checking. Hawthorn could ill afford to let him go if he had entered that room illegally. He motioned for the man to lead the way to the kitchen office.

Once inside the kitchen, the two men navigated their way around shelves and cutting tables, past the walk-in freezer, and through a small hallway that led back to the manager's office. The light was on and the blinds pulled shut. He knocked.

"Just a minute," a woman's voice called out. A moment later the door cracked opened. "Come in."

Dannette Marco sat near a computer with a pencil in one hand and a cup of coffee in the other. She was beautiful; a small turned-up nose perfectly centered between over-sized hazel eyes and curly locks of golden brown hair.

"Ms. Marco?" Jud stood quietly to Hawthorn's side with his hands crossed neatly in front of his lap.

Dannette gently placed her cup of coffee on the counter and swung a long pair of legs around the stool. "Yes, Dr. Hawthorn. What can I do for you?" Dannette motioned with her hands to ask him what he was doing. Her face was painted with question and concern.

Jud shrugged his shoulders.

"I'm sorry to bother you, Ms. Marco."

"Dannette, please," she said calmly.

Hawthorn cleared his throat. "Okay. Dannette. I found Mr. Parks here up on three."

"Yes. He delivered a plate to 349. Is there a problem?"

"What was the order?"

"Mashed potatoes and Jell-O, I think." She flashed some sign language to Jud who nodded. "Dr. Shane approved it. I've got his signature right here." She picked up a form from the countertop.

"Ms.- Dannette." Hawthorn took a deep breath, cupping his forehead with the palm of his hand. "Jesus. I apologize."

"Is everything all right, doctor?"

"Yes," Hawthorn answered. "Everything's fine." Hawthorn looked at Jud who appeared still confused by the conversation. "Please tell him I'm sorry."

"Sure."

Hawthorn walked quickly through the kitchen doors and into a hallway that connected the cafeteria to the main lobby. Once again he stood in front of the bronze elevator doors waiting for its arrival. He was relieved the worker was legit, but there was obviously a breakdown in Williams' security system.

Hawthorn stepped inside the elevator and pushed the button for the fifth floor. Just as the doors were about to shut a hand lodged itself between the panels. Hawthorn jumped.

"Sorry," a female voice called outside the door. The doors jolted open.

Struggling to enter was Cindy Powell, a bio-informatics researcher and lab technician for the CME. "Sorry, Hawthorn, I didn't know you were in here." She leaned over to pick up some computer equipment lying near her feet.

"No problem. You need help with that?" Hawthorn handed his charts to her and easily picked up the machine. "Where you headed?"

"Where I live," she replied, referring to the lab. He hit the button for the fourth floor and the elevator moved smoothly upward. Hawthorn had known Cindy since his first week at the Center. The two had even been romantically involved for a short while after his initial enrollment at the CME. Cindy was a down to earth, socially aware, environmentally sensitive woman. Though most male counterparts at the CME considered Cindy attractive, Hawthorn's primary magnetism to her was her loyal and trusting friendship. Her natural dedication to research was defined by lengthy hours spent examining the tiniest of details. In sharp contrast, Hawthorn's dreams would carry him in front of great and distinguished audiences around the world. Realizing their differences, the two parted as friends and never looked back.

"What's this for?" he asked.

"Extra power for that ADME-Tox module."

"Interesting," he said, inspecting the square housing. The back was open with multi-colored wires spilling out. The elevator stopped but the doors remained closed. Cindy reached into her shoulder bag and withdrew the silver access card, which she zipped through the vertical reader.

The doors quickly slid open, allowing the two to enter a darkened foyer. Directly before them was a set of huge steel doors. A halogen lamp in the back corner supplied the tiny room with a muted glow.

The research level was quite different from the others. The center of the floor was large and scattered with bits and pieces of machines and mechanical parts. The ceilings were twenty feet high and the length of the room fifty-five yards. This section of the research floor was for the machinists and inventors.

Lining each side of the large room were smaller research pods where individual doctors and researchers stored and worked on their projects in privacy. Each room had a unique locking system and there was no master key. Every time a doctor or researcher transferred, a new lock would be put in its place.

Rambling forward, Hawthorn passed the research pod where Mason kept his "memory mapping" device. The lights were off, the door shut, and the blinds on the windows tilted at the same angle he had seen them two days before. From here, he followed Cindy across the tiled floor to the back of the room. A large reflective sign above two doors read: NRA. Neuro-oncology Research Area.

Cindy approached the giant doorway and successfully completed the identical security routine with her magnetic card. This portion of the research area was much more orderly. Vials, expensive microscopes, and chemical incubators were stacked neatly against the walls. Stainless steel instruments and dishes lay in rows across sterile white countertops.

Cindy hit the lights. "You can put that over there." She motioned to a small table in the middle of the room.

Hawthorn lugged the machine to the table and carefully rested it on the flat surface.

Although Mason had vowed to continue MacMillan's private research, he'd since passed on some of the duties to Hawthorn who agreed to take the measurements for him on a bi-weekly basis. Hawthorn planned to record the numbers the next day but decided he may as well do it now while he was there.

"You haven't been here in a while, I noticed," Cindy remarked.

"I know, I know. Been pretty busy lately."

"I almost took the numbers for you."

Hawthorn walked over to a micro-refrigerator with a tiny padlock holding it shut. Similar to the research pods in the machinist area, each researcher here had their own equipment that only they could access. It was another of Williams' implementations designed to eliminate medical tampering.

"You talk to Mason lately?" Cindy asked.

"Sure. Why?"

"He was in here yesterday."

"Here?"

She nodded. "Said he needed to get some numbers."

Hawthorn looked over at his data log. Why would Mason need his numbers? This project had nothing to do with Mason anymore. Hawthorn scanned the log entries. There was no sign Mason had been there.

"No," she said. "He didn't look there. He was in the fridge. Moving things around. He had a key. I asked him what he was doing. Just mumbled something. You know how he is."

"Yeah," said Hawthorn, puzzled. Mason had a key but he never used it. Hawthorn opened the refrigeration unit and counted the tops of the vials. Each case looked full. All twenty-four were there.

"No ugly ducklings wandering off, huh?" Cindy asked.

"No. Everything's there." Hawthorn withdrew a vial and wrote down a number on his data log. When he was done, he replaced the vile and locked the door.

"Mason was here, huh?"

"Yeah. Didn't want to talk much, though. He seemed anxious. I don't know. I was busy, but he seemed to be rushing. Five minutes. Just clanking bottles around. Very hurried, though."

"Well, I'm sure he'll mention it later. No biggie."

"Nice to see you back in the lab."

"Don't get smart. Goodnight, Cindy."

Hawthorn moved briskly past the double steel doors and into the elevator. He was a half hour late. He retrieved the proper documents from his fifth floor office and sped off to Brenner's party.

CHAPTER EIGHT

Brenner's Swiss style mansion rested peacefully among towering firs and manicured grounds. In the distance was an Arabian stable centered on acres of tree-cleared, rolling land. The interior was equally grand; the living room and kitchen serving as a base for high-vaulted ceilings that apexed into an A-frame thirty-five feet overhead. Magnificent wooden beams stretched the length of the ceiling and beneath this dazzling display of structure, small groups of guests gabbed and circled a table full of food. House workers circulated through the room offering trays of hor'devours and glasses of Northern California's finest wine. From somewhere in the background, a slow piano riff rolled through the air.

Hawthorn stood with one of the head nurses in the far corner of the room gingerly sipping his drink. He looked at his watch, around the room, and then to his watch again.

"I'm surprised to see Dr. Xiao here. Aren't you?" she asked. Xiao was sitting alone on the stairs fighting through a piece of rolled meat. "From what I heard, Brenner had to practically beg him to join us."

"Doesn't surprise me."

"Oh, come on. He's not that bad. One of the other nurses sat down with him at lunch the other day. Of course, he didn't want her there, but she made him talk to her."

"I bet that was a stellar conversation," Hawthorn added.

"It was. Evidently he donates a lot of his time to working with children at the YMCA."

Hawthorn almost spit out his drink. "You've got to be kidding." Xiao was the last person Hawthorn would ever want around children.

"Serious. He spends his entire weekends working there."

"Incredible."

"Why do you say that?"

"Trust me, you don't want to know."

After moving through the food line, Hawthorn watched Xiao carry another plate back to the stairs nearby, where he continued to eat alone. Xiao didn't seem to mind keeping his distance from the rest of the group. He openly swore American physicians did nothing to understand his culture and, because of this, treated him as an outsider. He never did himself any favors as far as Hawthorn was concerned, so what the hell did he expect? He certainly enjoyed the American lifestyle, especially the benefits afforded to practicing physicians.

"Hello, Chen," Hawthorn said, forcing an uneasy conversation.

Xiao put down the rest of his lasagna and cleared his throat. "Hawthorn." Xiao wiped his mouth and took another sip of his drink.

Hawthorn really didn't know what more to say. The level of discomfort between them was enormous given the day's events. They had never publicly disagreed, but the fact that Xiao was Mason's main competition and Hawthorn a close friend lent itself to persistent discomfort.

"An unusual case this morning, wouldn't you agree?" Hawthorn asked, somewhat surprised at himself for going straight to the key topic.

"Yes. Tragic."

"Can you believe it was Alzheimer's? It didn't seem possible."

"If you're referring to Mason's diagnosis," Xiao commented matter-of-factly, "it was a wild shot in the dark. We still never answered the mortal question which is why that young girl is dead."

Hawthorn rolled his eyes. "What else is there to consider?"

"What or who?"

Hawthorn knew what Xiao was thinking and it pissed him off.

"If you want to know who I think killed her, I cannot say, although I do have my suspicions. If you want to know what killed her... well, I'm fairly certain of that."

Here it comes, Hawthorn thought.

"Negligence," Xiao said plainly. "Pure and simple." This was Xiao's strength. He could say whatever he wanted without the slightest bit of remorse or emotion and invariably he would end up under another person's skin. "Let's just say I'm considering ordering a second autopsy."

"What? Why? We just completed a thorough examination. It was inconclusive. What good is it going to do taking that young girl back to the table?"

"You forget, Hawthorn, that it is my sole responsibility to find answers for the family, for doctors, and for science. And-I-Am-Not-Satisfied."

"Perhaps you're taking your work too seriously. There's no reason to-"

"Death is a serious subject, Hawthorn. Especially when there is no reason for its existence." Xiao took another bite of his food and stared uninterested across the living room.

This was going nowhere. "Look, Chen, please reconsider. Mason did all he could."

Xiao sank his fork into the plate full of food. "Oh, I'm sure of that, Hawthorn. I am sure of that." He picked up his glass of wine and walked away, eventually finding a new spot where he could be alone to finish eating his meal.

*　　*　　*　　*　　*　　*　　*　　*

Across the room, Brenner conversed with a group of visiting physicians. From time to time she would instinctively scan the room, taking count of the conversations occurring outside of her own like a mother hen counting her chicks. Williams approached from behind, interrupting the conversation by placing a hand on her shoulder.

"Allen," she said, surprised to feel him close. "Let me introduce you to-"

"Sarah, can I have a word with you please?"

"Of course, Dr. Williams. Gentlemen, would you please excuse me?" Before she could set down her drink Williams pulled her, with his hand locked firmly on her elbow, to a vacant part of the room.

"What's this all about?" she asked lowering her voice. Brenner looked nervously around the room as if to make sure the other guests were not watching.

"Sarah, we talked about this."

"What?"

"How could you let Shane win the Brighton Award? You know damn well you're supposed to be investigating him, not praising him for a job well done."

She whipped her arm from his grasp.

"How could you let him win?"

"What are you talking about? You knew about it. That nomination was sent in long before- look, the fact that I headed the award nomination committee has nothing to do with-"

"But you *let* him win," he said.

"Listen Allen, I have done everything the Board of Directors has asked me to. Dr. Shane has done everything by the book."

"Would you listen to yourself, Sarah?" pleaded Williams. "His patients are dying."

"I understand that."

"Then would you please listen to what you're saying?"

"I know. I understand your concern. But there is no evidence of any wrongdoing. He has proven to be one of our finest doctors."

"Sarah. You weren't the one who had to face that young girl's grandmother and try to explain her death."

"Allen, I'm truly sorry but, again, I'm convinced that Dr. Shane is innocent thus far."

"Do you realize what is going to happen to the center if the press gets hold of the entire story including the award?" Brenner looked to the floor. "They'll tear us apart."

"We cannot accuse a doctor-"

"We are not accusing anyone," interrupted Williams. "But we do have to hold someone or something accountable for these two deaths sooner or later. And Mason was their doctor."

"Fine. But I refuse to implicate him without further investigation."

"I realize that, Sarah. Just don't let your personal feelings get in the way of this. I don't care how much his career means to you. I don't plan on placing the reputation of this entire institution on a physician who has lost two patients for no apparent reason. If you are trying to protect Dr. Shane's career by looking the other way, it will come at the expense of your own."

CHAPTER NINE

Through a wall of mammoth bay windows, Williams could see a steady drizzle falling softly on the outside deck. From time to time, an occasional gust of wind would blow pinecones and needles across the wooden floor. He hated being there. The chit-chat was killing him and the only reason he allowed himself this torture was to ensure Mason left with a positive attitude regarding the offer about to be made.

Inside, the party was finally quieting down. A couple of guests moved to and from a coffee maker located in one of the far corners of the open kitchen. Tables and countertops were now covered in leftover plates and empty wine glasses. Most of the riff-raff had left but many of the familiar doctors remained to finish out the evening.

Williams smiled. Mason approached. Showtime. "Our young star." He intercepted Mason a few yards away and steered him towards a vacant couch near the fireplace. "Mason, if I could please speak with you for just a moment."

Williams threw some pillows aside and, patting the top of a thick leather cushion, motioned for Mason to be seated next to him. Mason took a seat on the edge of the couch; elbows on his knees, shoulders rolled forward, eyes focused to the floor.

He finally had Mason alone. Williams' eyes poured over Mason like a fog, taking careful note of his obvious fatigue. The stress was wearing on him. "How is everything, Mason?"

"Okay."

Williams relaxed and leaned deeply into the cushions. "Well, that's nice. You deserve it. You've done well for both yourself and the center. I'm sure everything will return to normal, soon. These are just procedures, you know... standard policy."

Mason didn't answer.

Williams rocked himself forward. "Mason," he said in a more serious tone. "I have something to offer you. It's because of your recent accomplishments and this outstanding award."

Mason remained cautious, though his head turned slightly with interest.

"You see Mason, I've been in recent contact with a company named Geniomics. Have you heard of them?"

It was a rhetorical question. Williams knew Mason was familiar with their research. They'd been in the news almost every day.

"As you know, they're one of the leading research companies in the world. Of course they started out in high-tech, but they've built a strong financial base developing new techniques, new medicines, and... new machines."

Mason was listening now and Williams felt more in control of his presentation than he thought possible given the stakes involved.

"I happen to be close with their CEO. We've got some history together, one could say. He and I have set up a project that we would like to present to you. Now, remember, this is because we have the utmost confidence in your abilities."

"Dr. Williams, I don't-"

"Now wait a minute. I know the other opportunity I offered you was not that attractive. Certainly not for your caliber of work. That was my fault. Geniomics, however, would like to offer you something different... a collaboration of sorts, developing a new machine that would replace the existing MRI's."

Mason's eyes brightened notably. This was a project Mason originally put in front of the board in his first year of residency only to have it shot down by Williams himself.

"Are you serious?"

"Quite serious, Dr. Shane."

"And my current program?"

"You would probably have to put that on hold for a while. This project is expected to start immediately."

"And my practice?"

"Your job is secure. No need to worry about that. We'd get past the paperwork and you'd be on our way."

Williams could see Mason's brain already working on the design.

"Well, no rush, Mason. Think about it. But let me just tell you that the fellowship comes with a five hundred thousand dollar annual stipend. You can use it for whatever you want." Williams knew the money didn't matter. This was Mason's brainchild. As far as Williams was concerned, every one of these researchers was a mule and it was just a matter of dangling the right carrot in front of their myopic little worlds. "Can we touch base tomorrow?"

Mason nodded.

He patted Mason on the knee. "Perfect. I misjudged you and I am sorry about that. You're a special talent, Mason. Very special, indeed."

*   *   *   *   *   *   *   *

Hawthorn glanced outside. Glistening slashes of rain, illuminated by powerful outdoor lights, pounded the patio furniture and outside deck. Jordan, his fiancée, was an hour late. What the hell was she doing? Hawthorn rolled his eyes. He could only imagine what the excuse might be this time. Nothing new. He'd seen it before and it'd caused no less than a thousand arguments between them. Hawthorn was well aware he was born without the

patience gene but optional inefficiency killed him. Then
again, why she was late didn't matter. With this weather,
he was starting to get concerned.

With the storm gathering strength, the room's sole
illumination came from a large chandelier hanging above
the main room. Its pale yellow light provided the large and
airy room with a somber glow, softening the red leather
couches. Those who remained were locked in a focused
conversation. Even Xiao, standing at a distance behind the
makeshift circle, listened intently. Each doctor was
describing his or her most unusual medical story.

"You can't be serious, Dr. Rector," said Brenner.

BOOM.

A loud crack of thunder shook through the house.
The lights flickered.

"Apparently the youth decided to commit suicide by
hanging himself. He tied a rope to the ceiling, wrapped it
around his neck, and jumped off of the chair. Crazy thing
was, his weight wasn't enough to break his neck."

Rector wrapped his short fingers around his plump
neck as if to mimic the young boy's struggle. Pathologists
had a weird sense of humor. "Poor kid probably swung
there for minutes trying to free himself."

"Hank, that's horrible," said Brenner.

"I'm not kidding. Either his weight wasn't enough
or the chair was too small. But that's not it. When they
brought him in, he had these deep cuts on the inside of his
palms. Like a design or a picture. Intricate carvings. The
troubling thing was that the paramedics swore those
lacerations weren't there when they found him. The case
was absolutely frightening."

"Suicides rarely come off as planned," cracked Xiao
from afar.

The lights flickered again as Hawthorn glanced
outside. The rain was coming down hard. He felt both

angry and concerned. Perhaps he should call the Highway Patrol. Five more minutes.

"Did you ever consider the possibility that you may have encountered something spiritual?" Brenner asked.

"Sure. We thought about it."

"Oh please," interrupted Williams. "We're scientists, not monks. Don't try and tell me this young boy, while dead in the back of the van, carved some intricate design in his palms. Please. The paramedics must have overlooked something. It's the only plausible explanation."

Rector smiled. "That's it, though. We tested the lacerations. The burns around his neck occurred way before the lacerations on his hands. And he clearly died of asphyxiation. I'm sure of that. The cuts on his palms came sometime after. These things were like pictures. You know, crosses and circles. He would never have had time."

"Anything's possible," said Brenner. "Perhaps the medics were involved. Then again, who's to say what Hank witnessed that day wasn't a sign? What if there was something there?"

Williams crossed his arms disapprovingly. "Sarah, you know as well as I that lacerations are scientifically explainable."

"Plus, there was only one driver in this case," added Rector. "And the drive time from site to the center was normal."

A brilliant light filled the room causing the lights to flicker, struggle to regain, and then go out. The group waited silently in the dark for the lights to return but it appeared they were out for good. Hawthorn glanced quickly at the electrical devices as another bolt of lightening illuminated the room. Clocks. Microwave. VCR. All power was lost.

"That's getting close," Brenner said nervously. "We don't normally get storms like this. I'll get some candles."

Hawthorn had heard enough. He flipped the cover from his cell phone and noticed that there was still no signal. Frickin' PacBell. Those bastards were probably still locked in a game of cards next to the one cell tower needed to power his service. He had to do something. He walked towards the kitchen as Brenner returned with a box of matches and a lit a couple of candles.

"Anyway," continued Rector, "a year later the authorities found the same design in an attic of his father's house. Apparently his father was an artist. A painter who had passed on years before his son's death."

The rain swirled across the deck as powerful gusts diverted its downward path. Hawthorn picked up the receiver and clicked the lever several times to no avail. Jesus. He hung up the phone and checked his watch: 11:15.

BOOM. The lights flickered above and the room returned to darkness.

Hawthorn picked up the phone again and throttled the lever. His frustration was growing like a bad cancer. A hard rap sounded from the front door.

Hawthorn followed Brenner to the door as she used a candle to find her way into the foyer. She opened the door and stepped backwards to avoid the swirling rain.

"Hello. Sorry I'm late," Jordan said, closing an oversized umbrella.

Hawthorn shook his head and smiled. Out-punt the coverage, he thought, referring to the mismatch in looks between them. She was attractive with wavy blonde hair, high-arching brows, and long earrings that dangled jewels just off her neck. Although Hawthorn considered her far better looking and more sophisticated than he, she was also equally competitive and stubborn. This was especially evident in social situations. Sure, Hawthorn was likable and generally had no problem finding his way to the center of attention, but the way Jordan interacted with those around her was a piece of work. After all, Hawthorn had grown up commanding a mighty combine in the Texas heat while Jordan tipped champagne glasses round the world. The fact that her father was a legend on Wall Street afforded certain luxuries at a very young age: at twelve, a trip to Spain; at sixteen, a safari in Africa; and for her twentieth birthday, a tour of Russia.

This was in stark contrast to Hawthorn's life where each month employed creative financing to stave off an army of creditors. Regardless, it was her money and Hawthorn refused to take a cent of it.

Brenner helped remove a Donna Karan jacket and disappeared into the living room, leaving Jordan to drape her arms around Hawthorn's neck. "Hi, handsome," she said in a soft, sexy tone. "Did you get the dates?"

It'd been a month since they'd seen each other last. "Not yet," he answered. "I sent them in two weeks ago."

"John," she warned. "Tomorrow's the last day to book the flights."

"I know that. I'll take care of it tomorrow. I can't wait for that vacation." Hawthorn took her by the hand and led her back into the candlelit living room where the guests were again involved in a heated debate.

*　　*　　*　　*　　*　　*　　*　　*

Mason saw Hawthorn and Jordan enter the room from the foyer and seemed surprised that Hawthorn would be dating such a beautiful woman. It wasn't that Hawthorn was unattractive; on the contrary, many a hospital nurse had tried to befriend Mason to get to him.

What caught Mason's eye was something else. It was Jordan. As soon as Mason saw her, he felt uneasy. There was something about her. Perhaps they had met before. No. Mason was certain of that. A picture, maybe. No, not likely.

Mason stood.

"Jordan, I'd like you to meet Mason. Dr. Mason Shane," said Hawthorn.

Jordan smiled and extended her hand. "It's nice to finally meet you. John has told me so much about you."

Something in the eyes.

"Mason," said Hawthorn.

"Sorry, what?"

"It's nice to meet you, Dr. Shane," Jordan repeated, this time more slowly.

"Oh, uh... yes." He laughed. "It's- It's nice to meet you as well."

Her cheekbones, perhaps.

"Mason won the Brighton Award tonight," said Hawthorn. "It's very prestigious."

Jordan nodded politely. "That's wonderful. Congratulations."

"Thank you... I'm- I'm sorry. I feel a little-"

"Are you all right?" Hawthorn asked.

"Yes. I apologize. I'm truly sorry. Excuse me." Mason moved quickly towards the kitchen. He felt queasy. The room was beginning to spin. He veered to his right. He was light-headed.

BOOM. FLASH.

Mason was lost in a thick fog but seemed to be moving slowly forward. He extended his arm outwards to warn him of objects in his path and inhaled deeply. The air had no particular scent.

The mist soon faded and Mason realized he was located deep in an old-growth forest. Just ahead, a small, white-spotted deer grazed peacefully among several tall pines stretching high towards the afternoon sky. Beneath its tiny hooves was a lawn of crawling ferns that spread across the ground like a miniature canopy of trees. As the young doe ate from a tuft of grass, its darkened eyes scanned the silent facing of trees.

The deer scratched delicately at the ground and then lifted it's head to the sky as if to take in the mountain air through a pair of wide-open nostrils. All of a sudden, its ears apexed into small triangles. Each of its senses focused in one direction, its beady eyes frozen towards the tree line. Then the deer bolted into the safety of the forest, hopping and jumping over fallen trees and uneven rocks like a stone skipping through a pond. Thirty yards behind was a large, gray wolf closing fast for the kill.

The small doe bounced quickly through a narrow opening of trees and down into a small gully. The wolf paused and surveyed the landscape. In a matter of moments, it'd taken a different angle, moving speedily across the topside of a ridge where there were much fewer obstacles in its path. As the young deer struggled to make progress along the bottom of the narrowing ravine, the wolf jogged calmly along a twelve-foot ledge, keeping always a watchful eye on the laboring deer.

Finally, the young doe passed into a clearing where it could build speed and pull away from the wolf. From here it would escape into the expanding forest where its natural quickness and agility would prove its salvation.

Suddenly, the deer came to an immediate, sliding halt. From left to right the canyon walls were continuous. There were no more narrow openings through which the deer could escape. The canyon was boxed and its walls too steep for the small doe to climb.

The deer spun around and saw the wolf standing at the pinnacle of a large boulder. The wolf gave out a mighty howl that echoed throughout the forest as the doe backed up into the canyon's open jaws. Twenty yards away, the wolf broke into a full sprint. In a final cry for help, the small deer opened wide its blackened eyes and screamed a terrible noise.

BOOM.

Mason awoke, staring blankly up at the ceiling. A broken lamp and chair lay nearby. A thick bolt of lightening again filled the room.

"Mason, are you all right?" Hawthorn asked, shaking his arm. Other people were gathering around but Mason didn't recognize them. "Mason."

"Oh my God. Mason. Is he okay?" Brenner asked, overly concerned.

Mason squeezed his eyes shut and then opened them. He blinked a couple of times, looking around at the entire group. He stopped at Jordan and blinked again.

"I'd better go," he said softly. "I'm- I'm not feeling well."

"Jesus, what happened to you?" Hawthorn asked, helping him to his feet. Mason's first step caused him to stumble off-balance. Hawthorn steadied him with a hand on the shoulder.

"I'm just a little dizzy. I'd like to go home."

"Is he all right?" Brenner asked again.

"Probably a little too much celebrating," answered Hawthorn. "I'll take him home. He'll be fine."

Hawthorn carefully guided Mason to the door where Xiao sat amused at the bottom of the stairs. "Sticks and stones will break your bones..." he sneered.

*   *   *   *   *   *   *   *

Within minutes of starting the engine, Mason fell asleep against the closed window. For most of the ride home, Hawthorn divided his attention between the darkened roadway and Mason, making sure he was breathing normally and not experiencing any difficulties. He wanted to wake him to ask about his visit to the research lab. He wanted to know what Mason was looking for and why he hadn't mentioned anything. In the end,

Hawthorn figured Mason needed the sleep. The tremendous amount of pressure had obviously taken its toll.

A half hour later, Hawthorn pulled his car against the curb and helped Mason to his front door. He asked Mason if he wanted him to stay, but Mason assured him it was nothing. Dizziness, that's all.

As Hawthorn continued home, he reflected on the two patients who had mysteriously died. Hawthorn was surprised at the ease in which the hospital dealt with such a tragic situation. To his knowledge, there had been no formal investigation. The only thing that came close were the autopsies at which Mason was given a chance to speak confidentially among the other physicians.

Both Hawthorn and Jordan stayed awake for an hour sharing a cup of coffee and talking about what had occurred at Brenner's. For the most part, Hawthorn defended Mason, pointing to the fact that he was under a substantial amount of stress from the completion of his research project and the awards ceremony that night. He never said a word about the patients. She didn't need to hear it. It'd only worry her.

Laying in awake in bed, however, Hawthorn couldn't stop thinking about Mason. Something wasn't right. He could feel it in his stomach. Eventually he closed his eyes and planned his attack for the coming day.

DISCOVERY

CHAPTER TEN

Williams sat quietly in his office, his legs propped leisurely on the desk. A hot cup of coffee sat next to the phone steaming a marvelous aroma into the air. In one hand he held the remote control to a nearby television. In the other, Geniomics' annual report. He flipped the television on from across the room. Edmonds had been interviewed on 20/20 the previous night discussing the potential impact of their cold-curing drug on modern society.

The television framed Edmonds' face, his office serving as a sleek backdrop for the program. He appeared confident. Polished. Ready to fight.

"There are over 110 different forms of cold viruses and bacteria that have puzzled the medical arena since the beginning of mankind," explained the narrator. "So how has this rapidly growing company in the pacific Northwest found the answer? R2-X, as Geniomics calls it, uses a combination of synthetic and natural ingredients to attack and destroy the virus which initiates the common cold."

Williams fast-forwarded the tape. The report showed the Seattle factory. The R&D facilities in Bellevue. The pill. Edmond's face. Williams sipped his coffee and hit play.

"So what you're telling our viewers," said the reporter, "is that Geniomics is prepared to offer this drug on a world-wide basis at first launch. No regional roll-out."

Edmonds smiled. "That's correct. Extensive planning has gone into the preparation of this global event. Our company wants to be blind to international borders. Everyone around the world has the right to this cure."

"You've drawn some fire from your competitors on your plan to target business health plans as well. Are you concerned this may damage your reputation?"

"Not at all. Geniomics is a market-driven company and we are delivering exactly what the world wants. On average, a salaried employee suffers from respiratory viral infections at least once a year. If they're out of work for the day, that's eight hours they miss. At even twenty dollars per hour, that salaried person costs the company $160. What if you employ 10,000 workers? That's a million-six saved. Clearly, these businesses have an incentive to embrace our solution."

"I see."

"On the other end of the spectrum, what if you're a single mother working two jobs to make ends meet? Every single dollar counts. You can ill afford to not show up for work. Trust me. There is a market need for this every way we turn and we *will* deliver the cure. We're talking about affecting people's lives and the productivity of our nation's economy."

Williams turned off the VCR and dropped his legs beneath the desk. He watched from across the room as Mason cracked open the door and peered into his office. Finally, he would have an answer to the Geniomics offer. "Come in, Dr. Shane. Please."

Mason closed the door and walked the length of the room where he stood between two chairs facing the front of Williams' desk.

"Would you like something to drink?" Williams asked, fixing his posture. He folded his hands neatly on the desk.

"No thank you."

"Well then, how can I help you Dr. Shane? I trust you've given the Geniomics offer the proper thought?"

"Yes."

"Of course," said Dr. Williams. "A very prestigious offer."

"Yes, very."

Williams leaned forward as if he were about to tell a secret. "And very lucrative."

Mason smiled. "Sure. Lucrative. Yes."

Williams cocked back in his chair and threw his hands on top of his head. He felt relaxed. Certain.

"The truth is, Dr. Williams, I'm going to have to say 'no.'"

Williams smile turned immediately upside down as he brought himself quickly to the edge of his seat. "What?"

"I think the timing is wrong for me. I am committed to my own research. And since I'm nearing completion, I just think it's in my best interest to continue along the same path as before."

"Dr. Shane, are you crazy? This offer is the best career move you could possibly make. You've made it absolutely clear to everyone here that you are dedicated to pursuing neurological research. I have personally busted my back end to get the premier research company in the world to offer you this incredible opportunity. You'll call the shots."

"I understand and-"

Williams raised his voice. "No, Dr. Shane. I don't think you do. It would be foolish to turn down this offer. Absolutely. Perhaps you've not given it enough consideration."

"I have, Dr. Williams. I'm sorry. My decision is final. I appreciate your efforts. I do. I'm sure another researcher would love the opportunity."

Williams pounded one of his hands into an open fist. "Dr. Shane. I have set this up for you. For *you*. This will not be offered to anyone else in the world. Do you not understand that?"

Mason said nothing. He glanced outside.

"Why would you *ever* reject this opportunity?"

"Perhaps after I finish my current project."

"No. Of course, not. Look. I'm not the one with the money. The company's highest officials have made it painfully clear to me that if you wanted to take this opportunity with their company, you would be required to begin immediately."

"Then I'm truly sorry. Please tell them I'm honored by the opportunity. The timing is just not good right now. I apologize."

"Is that your final decision, Dr. Shane?" Williams' voice was turning harsh. He felt it unthinkable that Mason would be stupid enough to turn down this offer. Now what the hell was he going to do? Edmonds would kill him.

"Yes. It's final."

Williams' leaned back in his chair and closed his eyes. If he'd had a gun he would've killed Mason right there on the spot. And then himself. He'd never been fond of Mason or his selfish, martyr-like, pioneering attitude anyway. Mason was more like an arrogant punk whose name and ideas helped get a little publicity and some research dollars for the CME. And that was it. A complete circus show. Now, across two and a half feet of mahogany desktop, was this psycho screw-up whose devotion to his own work was about to impede Williams' path to a golden retirement. "Fine, Dr. Shane. I'll let them know. I hope you realize what you're doing. This is the chance of a lifetime."

Mason said nothing.

"That'll be all. Please leave."

Once Mason had closed the door, Williams turned on his computer and set up another communications link with Geniomics. Time was running out. The investigating committee was stalling, Mason had turned down the second offer, and to make matters worse, Edmonds would require a full and detailed explanation.

Williams fixed the camera and mike and cleared his throat. Again, the building's icons occupied the top half of his screen as Edmonds' image jerked slightly with each passing remark.

"Right on schedule," Edmonds beamed, this time a little lighter than the day before. Williams had promised Edmonds a link-up the minute Mason accepted the offer. "Give me the good news."

"He declined." Williams could see Edmonds' face turn suddenly angry as his fist swiped hard at the camera on top of his computer. The image went suddenly blank and ten seconds later Williams' phone was ringing.

"What do you mean he declined?" Edmonds barked. "You can't be serious."

"I'm very serious, Randy. He just left my office."

"Christ. My people have taken a full month to put this together for him. What was his reason?"

"Randy, are you sure we should be talking on this line?"

"I don't give a shit right now. You tell me why."

"He wants to finish his current project. We talked about this."

"And did you stress the money? Jesus, we more than doubled it over the first offer."

"Of course I told him. It made no difference."

"Damn't. What now, Allen? I'm over here kicking people's asses to pass these tests. The whole world thinks we've got these in the bag. Something's got to be done here."

"I know," Williams said, thinking.

"I mean soon. I don't have to tell you about the possible ramifications of failure on this."

"Of course not."

"Christ," Edmonds snapped. There was a long pause as both men searched for an answer. "This is unbelievable. What the hell is your committee doing? This guy's lost two patients."

"I don't know, Randy. They're trying to make sure they do things right. We should know something soon. Most likely today. I can try and get back to you later this afternoon."

"Allen, there is nothing I can do right now. It's entirely in your hands."

"I know. I know," said Williams. "I've got one more idea."

"Fine. Better be quick. Tick-tock, tick-tock, Mr. Williams. Tick-tock."

Williams pressed a three number code on his telephone.

"Yes, Dr. Williams." It was Nancy, his personal secretary.

"Get Dr. Rector in here right away. I need to talk to him as soon as possible."

"Yes, sir. Anything else?"

"No. That'll be all. Uh, wait."

"Yes?"

"Send Dr. Xiao in here as well. Separate meetings."

"I'll get right on that."

"Good." Williams disgustedly slammed the receiver into the phone's base and stared blankly across the room. After a few minutes he walked over to one of the counters and poured himself a fresh cup of coffee. DeCaf. Just as he was about to sit down, the phone rang.

"Williams here."

It was one of the assistants in Physical Therapy. A patient had just broken a $200,000 machine. Williams snapped loudly at him making sure that he find someone accountable. The assistant spouted assurances as Williams again slammed the phone onto the base.

He looked at the cup of coffee sitting on top of the counter. He was too sick to drink it. The phone rang again.

"What is it?" he cracked.

"Dr. Xiao is here as you requested."

"Fine. Send him in."

Xiao slid his way through the door and walked calmly to the front of Williams' desk. He was dressed in a white smock that was stained with a blur of reddish-yellow colors.

"You wanted to see me?"

Williams poured his cup of coffee into a nearby plant and walked around to the front of the desk. "Business attire as always, Dr. Xiao. Please. Sit," he said motioning to one of the chairs.

"I hope you found your way up here okay," Williams asked with a sarcastic smile.

"I'm happy you have faith in my navigation skills, Dr. Williams. What does this concern?"

"Let's talk about your recent work."

Xiao gazed reluctantly across the room. "Do we have to get into this again? I completed the last project flawlessly. I'm finished with that now."

"True. You performed your duty. So well, in fact, that I have another bit of research that calls for your 'flawless' skills."

"I really don't need this."

"Dr. Xiao, can you tell me when your work permit expires?" Xiao said nothing. He knew what that meant.

"That's better," Williams said with a slight grin. "Besides, I know you'll appreciate this new project. It's right up your alley. Full benefits."

"Can I leave now?" asked Xiao, somewhat disgusted.

"Yes. Of course." Xiao stood and made his way through the door. "I'll be in touch," called Williams. "I will definitely be in touch."

Thirty seconds later the door opened and Dr. Rector cautiously took a seat, his pudgy frame barely fitting between the armrests of the Victorian chair.

"Hank? It's no secret that as long as you remain devoted to the center, you'll be next in line for my post." Rector nodded enthusiastically. "You've done well so far, but there is still some work to be done. I have but one last little detail that needs some cleaning up before I hand you the throne."

CHAPTER ELEVEN

It wasn't even noon and Hawthorn had already experienced a full day of work. The morning began with a staff meeting covering critically important items like the theft of hospital gauze pads and the move to paperless forms. He would have easily fallen asleep had Cindy not ranted secretly about the social consequences of using differing algorithms during virtual high-throughput drug screening.

Hawthorn then visited the outpatient center to see one of his patients who had experienced side effects from the prescription drug Trifuluoperazine Hydrochloride. He'd prescribed the drug to help manage the manifestations of various psychotic disorders.

This particular patient had been in a freeway accident in which he suffered a severe skull fracture and some minor swelling of the upper spinal cord. After sleeping in a coma for nearly three weeks, he awoke to claim he'd been abducted for reproductive experimentation by a group of fat, roving beavers. As it turned out, he'd been treated before for mental instability and this fascination with beavers was no more than an ongoing saga in his mind.

At this point, however, it was a bit late for the standard treatment. The patient was giving the orderlies all they could handle so Hawthorn jumped in to help. One of the orderlies lost his grip on the patient's arm, which smacked Hawthorn to the ground.

After icing his mouth in the physician's lounge, he grabbed a quick lunch in the cafeteria with Cindy. Neither she nor Hawthorn had heard of any overt steps taken by the Center to resolve the controversy surrounding Mason's patients. A brief detective visit from the local station and more schedule restrictions were about all the other physicians and privileged staff had seen. Hawthorn voiced his intention of talking to Dr. Williams himself. How in the world did Williams expect a physician to perform well under such stressful conditions? It was beginning to affect Mason's mind and his work.

Hawthorn stepped confidently into the hallway of the third floor. He glanced at his clipboard. 302. Mr. Lewis. Hawthorn reacquainted himself with Mr. Lewis' condition. Middle-aged white male. Head injuries. Significant swelling in the frontal lobes.

Williams had requested that Mason assist Hawthorn with a number of patients due to his extensive knowledge on memory loss and recuperative therapy. This was the first day Mr. Lewis would not be heavily medicated which meant a much cleaner approach for the two young physicians. Hawthorn looked at his watch. Mason should be there by now.

Hawthorn entered the room to find Mr. Lewis alone, resting peacefully beneath a thin white sheet. A rotating fan in the corner of the small quarters served as the only rival to the sounds of a beeping pulse monitor. There were a few vases full of flowers near the window, but for the most part, the room was empty. A large monitor, just above the right side of the bed, displayed the patient's jagged vital signs in graphic form. Pulse. Breathing. Blood oxygen.

Hawthorn moved quietly around the end of the bed until he was within an arm's reach of the monitor. He looked over the vital sign indicators and then watched the patient's chest rise and fall. He looked again to his watch and then to the door.

Where the hell is he?

Hawthorn touched a small illuminated box on the monitor that was located beneath the various graphs. The

screen split instantly into two parts with the vital sign
graphs squeezed together in the upper portion and a new
series of touch-tone menus in the lower half. He tapped a
few more illuminated boxes in order to capture the various
readouts.

Mr. Lewis slowly opened his eyes, staring blankly
towards Hawthorn who finished resetting the machine.

"How you doing today, Mr. Lewis? I'm Dr.
Hawthorn. You're in the hospital. It's OK."

Mr. Lewis coughed.

"How are you feeling?" Hawthorn pulled a chair
alongside the bed and took a seat at its edge. He glanced at
his clipboard to review the other wounds Mr. Lewis had
sustained. Broken fibula.

"My leg hurts."

Hawthorn stood and leaned over the edge of the bed
placing his hands on the outer shell of the soft cast.
"There's really not much I can do at this point. You need
to let yourself heal."

"What happened?"

Mason opened the door and burst into the room. He
looked tired and irritable.

"Ah, just who I was looking for," said Hawthorn,
shooting a derisive stare across the bed. Mason tossed his
clipboard on a nearby table and forcefully slammed his
chair next to the mattress. "You'll have to ask Dr. Shane,
but I think you're making good progress."

Mason had yet to make eye contact with Hawthorn.

The patient winced as he twisted painfully towards
Mason. "Do you know what-"

"You were involved in a car accident. Your side of
the truck was completely destroyed."

Hawthorn was caught by surprise and raced to cover
Mason's ill-timed remark. "I'd say you were pretty lucky."
He glared at Mason from across the bed and then
continued. "Mr. Lewis has shown some major

improvements since our last check, Dr. Shane. It appears he still has mild trauma, but the fracture appears to be healing quite nicely. Everything else looks good."

Mason said nothing. He sat silently reading over the patient's case history. Hawthorn suddenly felt nervous. Mason was always prepared and could give an accurate diagnosis on the spot. His ability to recall the tiniest of details from a case history that could conceivably run hundreds of pages long was unique.

"Did you get that, Dr. Shane?"

"Yeah."

"Dr. Shane."

"I said I heard you, John," Mason snapped.

"And I said everything looks good."

Mason closed the blue cover of the case history and set it on the ground next to his seat. He rolled his chair to the end of Mr. Lewis' bed and began to palpate the skin around the wound on the patient's broken leg.

"Oww! Jesus!" cried Mr. Lewis. He looked to Hawthorn for help.

Mason pulled away from the leg and wrote something down on his clipboard. "There's new swelling around the wound."

"I didn't see-"

"There's no sense taking chances. Let's give the patient four hundred milligrams of Latafan intravenously."

"Four hundred?" Hawthorn asked, surprised. That was a bit excessive.

"And let's continue with the Morphine for the pain."

"Dr. Shane," said Hawthorn, firmly. "Can we speak outside?" Hawthorn questioned whether the Morphine was necessary. For the last few days, Mr. Lewis' condition had been improving rapidly. Not in a million years would Mason have prescribed Morphine at this stage.

"Well let's see, Dr. Hawthorn." Mason turned his attention towards the patient. "Are you in pain, sir?"

Mr. Lewis hesitated and then nodded his head.

"Well, Dr. Hawthorn here thinks we shouldn't give you anything for that."

"I never said that."

"Do you agree with that, Mr. Lewis?" The patient clearly disagreed. "Then it's all settled. We'll see you early Wednesday. You get some rest. Dr. Hawthorn, shall we?" Mason calmly held open the door.

The patient turned to Hawthorn looking for an answer, for trust. Hawthorn smiled. "You'll be fine. It's just a precaution."

As the two men entered the hallway to walk to the next room, Hawthorn grabbed Mason by the elbow and forced him into an unoccupied waiting room. "What the hell is wrong with you?" he whispered.

"John, really."

"Don't you talk to me like that. What in God's name is wrong with you today? You're not being a doctor. You fly in there late and practically start punching a patient's wound. Those are serious meds." As Hawthorn spoke, he looked nervously at the hallway, and then lowered his voice. "How do you think we're going to get an accurate picture of his condition if you don't let him off of that medication? It's been *five* days."

"Are you suggesting we not treat Mr. Lewis' pain?"

"Mason, I don't have the faintest notion of what's gotten into you, but these are my patients. Do you understand? *My* patients."

Mason lowered his head as if he suddenly understood his brashness. He became instantly deflated. "I know, Hawthorn. I apologize."

"What's with you? Huh?"

"I didn't sleep last night. I'm having-"

"Well, you don't take it out on our patients. Especially my patients."

"You're right. You're right. I'm sorry."

"What the hell happened to you last night? If you're having problems, you need to get checked out. You're not doing anyone any good here."

"I don't know, John. Some strange things have been happening lately."

"Like what? More headaches?"

"It's nothing, I'll stop by neurology later today."

"What things?"

Mason sighed and looked out into the hallway. "I'm having visions, John. Crazy things that don't make sense." He looked sternly into Hawthorn's eyes. "I want you to hook me up."

Hawthorn's expression narrowed with apprehension. "No way, Mason. We've talked a hundred times about that. You promised never to get involved with it."

"Hawthorn, something is going on here. I'm getting glimpses of something - like a story being told only I get one scene at a time and so none of them make sense. I'm blacking out for hours at a time, I throw up six times a day, and to top it off, my patients are dying. I need a second person there and you're the only one I can trust. You're the only one who knows how to operate it."

Hawthorn was stunned. He had no idea Mason's nerves were causing him such physical harm. "I can't, Mason. I just can't. What if something went wrong?"

"Nothing will go wrong."

"What if something did? I couldn't live with it. Just so you can explore your own dreams?"

"They're not dreams, John."

"No way," Hawthorn answered. "I won't. That's it. Please don't ask me again. I'd really like for you to go up to Neurology. Give them a chance."

Mason stared at Hawthorn for a long moment and then said, "Fine."

"Do you want me to come with you?"

"No. I'm fine."

Hawthorn remained upbeat to mask his concern. "You've been working yourself pretty hard lately. Maybe you should take a break. Dinner?"

"I can't. I'm fine, Hawthorn. Let's go."

"If we work too much, we'll both go crazy," said Hawthorn.

Within seconds they were at the next patient's room. 363. Mr. Boles Johnson. Bolley, as the nurses called him, was a sixty-two year old African-American whose Louis Armstrong voice filled the hallways every morning at 7 a.m.

Bolley had experienced a major heart attack a week before and was having some final tests performed before his release. There was concern that a blood clot could develop near his brain, so the General Surgeon asked both Mason and Hawthorn to monitor the patient's blood volume until he could be cleared for release.

Bolley's room was filled with flowers, cards, and pictures of his grandchildren. Thirty-five in all. Ten great grand kids. Balloons covered with 'Get Well' messages floated high above every corner of the room.

"Look what the cat drug in," Bolley said, smiling from ear to ear. "I thought we were through goofing around here. This ticker's going another round."

"Morning, Mr. Johnson. Looks like you'll be free to go soon."

"How soon? I might want to stay. Some pretty young ladies floatin 'round here."

Mason adjusted his IV and the men said their goodbyes.

"That guy is great," said Hawthorn, the two men again traveling down the hallway. "Why can't all patients-"

"He'll be dead by the end of the week."

"What?"

"His cholesterol level is the highest I've ever seen. His EEG indicated the presence of an arrhythmic pulse. His arteries are probably seventy percent blocked. Maybe eighty. And that was three days ago. What the hell is Gordan thinking?"

Dr. Thomas Gordan was the General Surgeon who had control over most patients leaving the Intensive Care Unit. Hawthorn knew the man to be warm and gentle with his patients. About four years ago he misdiagnosed a patient's condition that may have contributed to his death. It was largely rumored that since he was a close friend of Williams', the hospital covered his mistake through a barrage of suspect documentation. In other words, it was difficult to envision him making any more mistakes.

"Seventy percent? You can't be serious."

"I am. Gordan won't authorize Warifan. What is he thinking? We need to thin his blood."

"He's a hemophiliac, Mason. What do you expect? You can't thin his blood."

Mason stopped. "That man's life is about to come to a halt if we don't do something. His arteries are clogging at a rapid pace and that, my friend, is fatal. Would you rather save his life now and worry about complications, or let him go?"

Hawthorn was surprised at Mason's directness. "Have you tried talking to Gordan?"

"Of course," Mason answered, walking again. "He's avoiding me. He's not returning my calls or emails. I've been by his office a hundred times."

"He did ask us to monitor Mr. Johnson's blood volume through the MRI. Technically, he still has authority on pulmonary decisions."

"This is bullshit."

"Dr. Shane!" Williams was stomping his way down the hall towards them. He appeared extremely agitated. "Dr. Shane, can I have a word with you?"

"Of course, Dr. Williams," Mason replied.

"Dr. Shane, I have a serious complaint from one of your patients. It appears your diagnosis frightened her quite badly. I personally had to reassure her."

"Was I in error, doctor?" Mason asked.

"No, but that's not the point. There are two roles that a doctor must perform. Diagnosing an illness is an important skill but you should never forget that you are dealing with a human being."

"Should I have lied to her?"

Mason's indifference was fueling Williams' frustration. "That is not what I am saying. And you know it. Doctors are not gods. You should know when it is just as important to comfort a patient as to cure them."

"I understand, Dr. Williams, but my primary interest is in research."

"There is no excuse for your behavior today."

"It was important to be honest with her."

"For God sakes. You have to be sensitive to each situation. Telling someone that they have Multiple Sclerosis is never easy, but you could have shown some compassion."

"I'm sorry, doctor. I'm not feeling well today."

"That's pathetic," Williams said in near disbelief. "That patient's life is over as she knows it and you're telling me you're having a bad day?"

Mason fell silent.

"You're skating on thin ice, here, Mason. Thin ice on a very warm day." Williams stormed away apparently satisfied with his attack.

"You better be careful, Mason," Hawthorn warned.

"I know that. But last night he-"

Mason suddenly appeared dizzy. His knees buckled slightly as he veered sideways towards the wall. Hawthorn grabbed him quickly by the forearm. "Jesus, Mason. What's wrong with you?"

"I- I really don't know." He inhaled deeply. "Wow." He breathed deeply again.

"Why don't you go up to Neurology now. Then go on home. I'll cover."

Mason looked up and down the hallway. "I think I just need to lie down."

"Go, Mason. I got it. I'll call you for dinner if you feel up to it. Take a nap or something."

As Hawthorn watched Mason weave his way through the circus-like atmosphere of the third floor, he tried to put himself in Mason's shoes. For the past few months Mason had poured his heart and soul into that research. With the ICC and FDA approvals not far away, his research would not only treat Alzheimer's and amnesia but could also enhance memory recollection, which meant advanced and possibly expeditious learning for the average human being. The ramifications of Mason's invention were endless. It was a breakthrough that could very well facilitate future discoveries and advancements for the entire human race. And here was Mason, caught between the excitement of earth-shaking research and the uncertainty of lives beneath his wing. It was clear that the stress surrounding his job was taking a toll on his judgment and his health.

Hawthorn tried to think of a way to help. He'd always stood up for the underdog. He'd always been there for friends in need. Who did Mason have to lean on? He had no family.

He needed to do something. Williams had misinterpreted Mason's actions. After all, Mason was under tremendous pressure and stress. Screaming at a physician who had inexplicably lost two patients was not the best thing for improving his performance. Perhaps a little consideration from a concerned third party would help smooth things over.

Sweeping through the fifth-floor hallway, Hawthorn snatched a small sunflower from a vase on a nearby table and quickly found his way to Williams' office at the far end of the hall.

"Where's the party girl?" Hawthorn asked, popping into the receptionist area. He held out the flower. Both he and Williams' secretary, Nancy Hoyt, had once been severely inebriated together at a physician get-together. Ever since, they continued to joke about the night's theatrical antics.

Hawthorn's smile disappeared. There was no one there. At first he figured she might have left early for the day, but Williams would never have allowed that. Besides, all of her papers were still strewn about her desk and the cover had not yet been placed on her computer. Some steam rose from a nearby pot of tea.

He took three cautious steps forward and paused at the front of Nancy's desk, glancing over the swarm of papers and envelopes. He walked back to the doorway, opened it, and stared down the long vacant hall. There was no sign of her.

Hawthorn retreated and again looked over the vacant room trying to decide what to do. All of the courage mustered to confront Dr. Williams was fading. He thought about leaving but then remembered that Williams had promised the new schedule would be available that afternoon. Hawthorn looked again across Nancy's desk for the familiar form. Today was the last day to book his flights. There was no way he could afford the regular price.

Hawthorn walked quietly over to William's door and listened. He couldn't tell whether Williams was in there or not.

After doling out three quick raps against the closed door, Hawthorn cleared his throat and tucked in his shirt, making sure to flatten each and every embarrassing crease. He waited nervously for an answer and then gave three more light raps against the solid wood door. Perhaps Williams was in a meeting or on the phone. Hawthorn thought about leaving but then paused. He needed those dates. He carefully placed his hand on the doorknob and gave it a slow, cautious turn.

Click.

Hawthorn peeked his head through the crack and saw that Williams' office was abandoned as well. From across the room he could see the magnificent view that served as the backdrop for Williams' desk. Treetops for miles.

Hawthorn stepped back and was about to close the door when he noticed some documents sitting on Williams' desk. *The schedule.* He hesitated, then slipped inside.

Hawthorn spun quickly around the side of Williams' desk and flipped over the first document. An invoice. More invoices. A green light was flashing on the computer. The monitor was off but the computer was on. Hawthorn glanced at the back of the door. Screw it. He needed that info.

A quick flash and the screen suddenly came to life. As Hawthorn kept his nervous sight balanced between the door and the computer, the blackened screen slowly gave way to perceivable message. 'PRINT FINISHED'. Hawthorn scanned the room and quickly located the printer along the far wall. In its cache were two freshly printed pages.

Hawthorn turned off the monitor and moved speedily to the printer where he flipped over the first sheet of paper. It was a printout of an email from Williams, clearly not the schedule.

As he placed the sheet back onto the tray, a familiar name caught his eye: Dr. Mason Shane. Hawthorn glanced again to the closed door and then to the paper. It was none of his business. He sat the document in the tray.

Then again, it was his business. Mason was a close friend and a lot of strange things had been happening to him over the past few weeks. Maybe this could shed some light on what the hospital was doing to resolve this nightmare of a situation.

From: Awilliams@cme.org
Re: Research Opportunity, Dr. Mason Shane

At this point the information meant nothing. As far as Hawthorn knew, Mason received at least two or three of these a week.

A small tap at the door froze Hawthorn. He could see the handle being turned. He was caught. Hawthorn dropped the paper back into the bin and straightened his posture into something he felt looked natural.

"Hello?" a man's voice called into the room. A narrow-faced man in wire-rimmed glasses peered his head around the corner. He appeared to be wearing a uniform of some sort.

"Hello?" he called again.

Hawthorn cleared his throat. "Yes? Can I help you?"

The young man stepped into the room. UPS.

"I have a package for a..." He looked down on his electronic clipboard. "Dr. Allen Williams?"

"I'm afraid he's not available right now."

"Is this your office?" the man asked, fidgeting with his glasses.

"Uh, no. No it isn't. This is Dr. Williams' office."

"Oh, that's all right, I just need someone to sign for it. I'll just set this down right here." He placed the package beneath an antique desk in the corner of the room and then walked over to Hawthorn holding out the clipboard. A metallic pen swung freely by a string. Hawthorn quickly signed his name.

"Did you press hard?" the man asked, looking over the signature. "Sometimes these things don't register. Well, you have a good day now."

Hawthorn nodded as the UPS man walked towards the door. After a few steps he paused and spun around. "Oh, I almost forgot. Here's his mail. I've ran into that same postman five times already today. Can you believe it?"

Hawthorn didn't want to speak. He followed him to the door making sure the man had exited the area completely. Satisfied, he quickly made his way back to the printer where he frantically skimmed the letter.

Randy,

Will contact you early tomorrow to discuss. At this time, he refuses to accept the offer. Perhaps we should increase to $1,000,000/ yr. Something to think about.

A.

PS. No change in Sam's condition.

Hawthorn was shocked. He could hardly believe it. Mason hadn't mentioned anything to him about a grant, especially one for that amount. One million dollars? Hawthorn would do just about anything for that kind of money. Most of Mason's offers were around two hundred thousand. Maybe two and a half. But this was unbelievable. He scanned the page for the name of the sponsor. Who the hell was the company? And who was Sam? It didn't make sense.

Hawthorn quickly placed the two sheets back into their original position. He paused next to a nearby table and curiously browsed through the six mail envelopes just delivered:

ZaniCon Corp.
13543 W. 39th
New York City, NY 10017

Beldat Inc.
917 N. Camderdon St.
Los Angeles, CA 90064

Patricia S. Mullin
4545 Meade Ln.
Castle Hill, CO 80205

Geniomics Inc.
2222 W. 79th Ave.
Seattle, WA 98101

Karen Smith
815 Lavar Lane
Flagstaff, AZ 86001

Samuel A. Klinger
900 W. Ben Kate St.,
St. Louis, MO 63108

He figured Mason would know what he was talking about, but he had no idea who would have offered that kind of money. Not even the big guys. Perhaps it was a private donor.

Hawthorn slipped into the reception area and grabbed the door's handle to enter the hallway. Suddenly, he paused. Somewhere down the hall he could hear a man's voice getting louder and louder. *Williams.* Hawthorn sat quickly on the couch as the door flew open.

"I'm telling you, I just don't agree with the way those idiots are handling it," Williams sounded. Nancy followed closely behind with pen and paper in hand.

"I think- Dr. Hawthorn, what are you doing here?" Nancy gave a quick smile and a wave.

Hawthorn stood. "I wanted to discuss my vacation plans."

"Vacation? What vacation?" Williams was screwing with him. Hawthorn played along and threw him a fake smile.

"We talked about a one week leave. Last month."

"Hmmm. I just don't remem- oh, yes, to Mexico I remember."

"No sir. It was the Caribbean."

"Uh-huh," Williams said with extreme unimportance. He was busy looking over a document in his hands. "I think something can be worked out. As a matter of fact, I do believe I've allowed you this leave."

Williams tossed the packet of papers onto Nancy's desk. He picked up his own clipboard and flipped through a couple of pages. "Yes, Dr. Hawthorn, you're cleared through the 22nd."

"Thank you, Dr. Williams. I was also hoping to-"

Williams ignored him, entered his office and shut the door. Although Hawthorn desperately wanted to speak on Mason's behalf, he figured it wasn't worth it to try and recapture Williams' attention. Especially after that brief whim of benevolence.

"A vacation?" asked Nancy. She was a petite woman, oval in stature and slightly overweight. She'd worked with Dr. William's for nearly twenty years. She had a pleasant way about her; her kindness was renowned throughout the Center. She'd do anything for anybody, anytime. More important, perhaps, was that the other physicians knew she was the only person whom Williams would listen to; his eyes and ears to the world.

Hawthorn nodded. "An anniversary of sorts."

"Well, that sounds splendid. Same lucky girl? You know how jealous older women can be." She winked but her smile was short-lived.

Hawthorn put his hands on the edge of her desk leaning deliberately towards her. His voice was low and urgent. "Can you get me a copy of Mason's X-report?"

Nancy's mouth opened slightly, surprised by Hawthorn's words. An X-report was a confidential investigative file drafted by Williams' own security team, which incorporated the police report as well as their own internal investigation of how the Center's security infrastructure performed in various events. Hawthorn had heard of its existence from a former staff member who was wrongly accused and terminated. He wasn't sure if one existed in this case but it was worth fishing for.

Nancy was thrown off-guard. "Wha... you mean from earlier this-"

Hawthorn nodded as he glanced nervously towards Williams' door. He'd found an angle.

"Oh, uh, geez, Hawthorn, I don't know." She was already shaking her head. "No. I could get in a lot of trouble."

"Nancy," he whispered, "I would never ask you to do this if I didn't think it was important. Mason's in trouble. You know that. I just think that maybe..." He paused wondering if he should go further or just leave. "I just want to make sure nothing was overlooked."

"Like what? Nobody knows what happened. The poli-"

Hawthorn placed a finger on his mouth reminding her to lower her voice. "I don't know. Something seems... something's wrong here."

Nancy's eyes scanned the top of her desk, thinking. She was close to turning. Hawthorn knew she wanted to help, but if Williams discovered that this information was leaked, Nancy would be fired for sure.

"I need that report as a basis to start looking. Please," Hawthorn appealed. "I know that committee is looking into it, but I just can't see him- Look, all I need is an hour. You can trust me."

"Fine," she answered, glancing at Williams' door. "You mean-"

"I'll leave a copy with Howard. Now please leave. And Hawthorn," she said quietly. "Not a word."

He gave her the flower and mouthed the words 'thank you'. He had ten minutes to get to the travel agent and purchase the tickets. Afterwards, he would head home to prepare himself for dinner with Mason. Hopefully a half-day's rest would help clear Mason's cobwebs.

CHAPTER TWELVE

From the hospital, Mason traveled directly to the
Old County Library where he spent an hour or two
reviewing medical journals and books on dream
interpretations and psychic phenomenon. The Old County
Library was an off-white, limestone building with huge
Dorian pillars and an impressive staircase entry. The
interior was adorned with high-back King's chairs
anchoring large oak tables. The original bookcases were
ten feet tall and cradled the library's assets old and new.
Built in the late 1800's by a wealthy gold miner and his
family, the library was now supported by several private
grants and endowment chairs. Over time, the institution
had assembled a collection of scientific materials that
rivaled the local university archives.

Mason had exhausted the available content at the
CME and nothing provided the answer he was looking for.
The doctors in neurology offered little explanation for his
blackouts and visions, only that they needed to run
additional tests. Frustrated further, he left the library and
continued home.

Mason turned a book over in his lap and squeezed
shut his eyes which burned from exhaustion. He thought
about the girl, Myra, and then the young boy. What could
he have missed? The clock above his television informed
him he'd been sitting in the same position, a worn out
recliner in the middle of his living room, for the past three
hours. He hardly remembered sitting down.

Between the pages of the book, Mason withdrew a
small black and white photograph of him and his
grandfather. The two stood proudly in front of a lone
trading post somewhere on the reservation. A sunken-

chested boy with bony white legs, Mason held a large feather in his hands and posed proudly next to the elderly man.

Mason stared deeply into the picture. He felt detached. Empty. Outside, a swirling breeze rang a set of wind chimes.

BOOM. FLASH.

Mason was lost in a beautiful bright light. Panicked at first, his fear quickly melted into wonder as the light faded and Mason recognized the small hogan in which he lived with his grandfather on the arid reservation.

The land around him was flat and dry with an occasional desert plant pocking the reddish-brown soil. Deep shades of blue filled the overhead sky as the afternoon sun bore down heavily upon the hot desert floor. Marble-colored cliffs framed the horizon's edge in nearly every direction.

Mason's grandfather sat on a small wooden bench beneath the shaded edge of the hogan's flat stone roof. His long gray hair and weathered face bespoke of a man who'd endured the wrath of time. It'd been over ten years since his grandfather's death and to his deepest regret, Mason was never given the chance to say good-bye. His grandfather had suffered a stroke at a distant water hole while Mason stayed behind to practice his studies.

Mason tried to step forward but found that his position was fixed. He looked all around but there was no trace of his bodily existence. There were no shadows cast and no sounds to be heard. It was as if someone had suspended a camera in mid-air. Frustrated, he screamed. "Grandpa!"

His voice echoed loudly through the valley but there was no sign that the old man could hear him. A set of clay wind chimes rang loudly beneath the hogan's roof.

A young, anglo-looking boy, eleven years of age, exited through the front door carrying an Eagle's feather. It was *him*. He appeared to be pouting in some childish way as he walked over to a small chair at the far end of the porch. The boy plopped down and closely examined the large feather in his hands.

"Mason, come," his grandfather said. Mason stared out at the desert, refusing to cooperate. "Do you know where that feather comes from?"

The young Mason stood and regarded the feather with both hands, turning it over and over. Occasionally he would run his fingers over the individual stalks.

"There once was a mother Eagle who lived high up in the cliffs above this valley." The young Mason glanced into the distance at the reddish-gray canyon walls. "One day she decided to teach her baby eagle how to fly. But a great storm rose in the west, and the mother Eagle and her baby soon found themselves battling the driving wind and rain."

"They fought as hard as they could but the baby soon grew tired. So the mother Eagle took her own feather and gave it to her son so that he could fly safely back to the nest."

The young Mason stood silently contemplating the story. He gave the feather one last rub and looked out into the desert. "Eagles can't share feathers." Nothing got past him.

His grandfather smiled and motioned for him to sit on his lap. Mason hopped up on his grandfather's knee. "No, but mothers love their sons."

"Why did my mother go away?" Mason asked.

"Sometimes a person may not be able to fight the dark spirit. There is no way to know when or why the Bearcloud will come, but always he brings misery."

His grandfather spun Mason between his legs and turned him around so that he could look deep into the young boy's eyes. "Your mother loved you, Mason, but when the Bearcloud came, she could not resist so he had to take her away."

"Will Bearcloud come for me, grandpa?"

Grandfather paused and took the feather from Mason's hands, straightening the stalks with his own weathered fingers. "So long as you are with me, Little Wolf, you shall be protected."

Grandfather handed the feather back to the boy and Mason gave him a long hug.

BOOM.

Mason slowly opened his eyes taking a moment to gather himself. He was still seated in the same position with the photo lodged between his two hands. Another two hours had passed.

Mason withdrew one of his hands from the photograph and wiped clean a streaking tear from his face. For a short while he stared closely at the tiny drop of water that sat obediently at the tip of his finger as if he were about to lose a priceless memory.

The phone rang loudly. Mason glanced at an antique clock pinned to one of the walls: 6:18 p.m. He thought about not attending Hawthorn's dinner invitation. He didn't feel like talking anymore. He wanted to sleep.

Mason leaned over the edge of the chair and picked up a small bottle of unmarked pills. He spun the bottle around and around, considering their contents. The phone stopped ringing and then started up again. Mason popped the top and poured a couple into his hand. He looked down at the picture. His mind was trying to communicate. But what? A wolf, deer, eagle feathers, grandpa? He looked again to the pills. The first ones he'd taken two days ago had done nothing to bring meaning to the situation. Perhaps these three would be the answer. Finally, he opened wide and swallowed them whole.

In the background, he could hear the answering machine pick up. "Mason, Dr. Williams. Call me as soon as possible. This is urgent and simply cannot wait."

CHAPTER THIRTEEN

Giordano's was a Italian restaurant located in the historic district at the corner of Burnside and NW 11th Avenue. The restaurant's dimly lit interior was famous for its red velvety walls that were usually decorated with the works of a well-known, contemporary artist. The booth outlining the main floor were shaped in wide semi-circles and designed in a classic Victorian style with high arching backs and shiny gold beads accenting the seams.

It was eight thirty and Mason still hadn't shown. Hawthorn had politely asked the waiter to return at least six times and finally they'd decided to order for him.

"This place is great," Jordan said, watching the staff dart between the tables and the kitchen. "The colors are so vibrant."

Hawthorn smiled. "You know, it amazes me just how beautiful you are."

"It wouldn't amaze you if you took more time to visit me."

"Now, why would you say that? I just gave you a compliment for God's sakes."

"You were supposed to come to New Haven last week. It's been two months, John."

Hawthorn leaned back against the leather cushions of the booth. "Jordan, come on. This is the only the third time you've been out here to visit. If we're not meeting half-way every time, it's me traveling to Connecticut."

"That's not fair, John. You know I have the money."

"I know that. But you know how busy I've been. We've talked about this a thousand times. My schedule is extremely demanding right now. Do you have any idea what an average day is like for me?"

"Oh, please. It's not like you're the Secretary of State, John. You're a doctor. There are other things in life besides your career. You're the one that told me to remind you if you ever got too serious. Well, guess what, John? You're too serious."

"Jordan." He rested his palm on top of her hand. "Once you finish school we'll have the rest of our lives together. I promise things will die down. Right now I just have to focus hard and finish this thing out. It's almost over."

Jordan's look of concern gave way to a defeated smile that he'd come to know as her way of showing both warning and admiration for his focus and determination. "John, there's something important I think we should talk about. John?"

Mason was making his way around the maze of tables towards the booth.

"Apologies, I didn't realize…" Mason's words tapered as if he was under the impression that only he and Hawthorn would be dining alone.

Hawthorn scooted into the middle of the curved booth allowing Mason to be seated. He carried with him a walking stick his grandfather had carved for him when he was a young boy. From time to time he would use it to walk around the hospital giving the patients something new and interesting to see.

"It's okay," said Hawthorn. "We ordered for you. Hope you don't mind."

"Of course not," he replied. "I was tied up-"

"Don't worry about it, Mason. We were just talking about how busy the hospital keeps us."

For the next few minutes, Hawthorn tried anything to get Mason engaged in conversation. It was both impossible and frustrating. Mason appeared noticeably uncomfortable. Hawthorn glanced across the table at Jordan for help.

"Are you feeling a little better?" asked Jordan.

"Oh, yes. I was just a little... I just wasn't feeling well."

"Mason lost a-" Hawthorn caught himself before he could finish and then looked at Mason apologetically. He was so used to telling Jordan everything. It was automatic. Mason shook his head and motioned with his finger. "It's quite all right, Hawthorn. Go on."

"No. I'm so sorry."

"It happens," he said, his eyes fixed on a glass of water in front of him. "I lost a patient the other day and no one knows why."

A waiter approached with their food and for the next fifteen minutes Hawthorn tried to maintain Mason's involvement in conversation. Nothing worked. He was totally removed.

Hawthorn whipped a buzzing pager from his belt and looked wearily into the display. "It's ER." He nudged Mason from his seat and gathered an overcoat into his arms. "I'm really sorry about this."

"Let me take it, John" said Mason. "I need to get back anyway."

"Mason, relax. You're in good hands. It's my patient. I have to go. You two enjoy dinner. Get to know each other." Hawthorn put on his jacket and gave Jordan a kiss on the forehead. She looked up at him with a stern, greatly dissatisfied look. He'd done this to her the last time she was here. "I'm sorry. I'll make it up to you."

Hawthorn had barely left the table when he realized that he'd forgotten to ask Mason about the offer. "Mason, I almost forgot-" The pager buzzed again in his hand. "Never mind," he said. "I'll talk to you later."

*   *   *   *   *   *   *   *

Jordan watched Hawthorn exit the building. She was tempted to leave. What was he thinking? Mason had offered to take it. When was he going to put her ahead of some patient with a bellyache? And to leave her with some guy who's obviously having issues?

She looked across the table at Mason who remained fixated on his plate, slowly cutting a piece of ravioli. What must it feel like to lose a patient, she thought. Dreadful. She supposed the knowledge that the next one could be saved was what kept these guys moving. But Mason was peculiar. Supposedly brilliant, but how alone he must feel. She felt sorry for him in a way. "So what do you think about this place?"

"Never cared much for it."

"Yeah?"

"Yeah," he said, looking up at her for only a moment. "It's overdone. Food's okay but this is Portland."

"I know," she said. "I feel the same way. I'd never tell John that but I know what you mean. He just loves these places."

Jordan reached for her glass and saw the cane lying beside Mason on the bench. "Interesting cane you have there." It was made of pine and had unusual carvings up and down the stem. At the top was the hand piece, the head of a wolf. "Where'd you get it?"

Mason set down his fork and laid the cane across the table. "My grandfather carved it for me when I was fourteen. Said it was a symbol of strength, intellect, and bravery. Signified my passage from child to man."

"It's beautiful. Your grandfather must have been someone special."

"Yes," answered Mason. "He helped me find peace."

*   *   *   *   *   *   *   *

Mason rotated the cane in his hand. It'd been almost eighteen years ago to the day. He could never remember it all, but what he could remember was, at best, the worst picture he could ever imagine.

Mason had walked nearly two miles from school along a wet two-lane highway. Although the rain had diminished to an almost non-existent drizzle, the sky overhead was solid gray and appeared to be regaining its might. He left the main road and walked freely down a pothole-ridden dirt driveway, taking extra time to stomp in any puddle that got in his way.

As he approached the front door of a doublewide manufactured home, Mason could hear the sounds of two people yelling. His pace slowed. He'd heard them argue before but never like this. Occasionally, he could hear glass shattering against a wall or the floor.

Mason entered the tiny living room and quietly placed his backpack and lunch pail on a nearby chair. He walked cautiously towards the kitchen and peeked the round of his face beyond the corner of the door.

Smash.

A tall pitcher exploded near Mason's hand sending fragments of glass into his arm. He jerked away, and without making a sound, removed the small bits from his punctured skin.

"I don't need to hear your crap," his father yelled. "You can't stop drinking. Why can't you see that? You need help. I can't take it anymore."

Mason looked again into the kitchen. His mother crumpled into a protective ball next to the refrigerator as his father whirled glasses and plates above her head.

"Every day I come here and have to listen to you bitch. Every single day I clean up the mess, my- my drunk wife has made. What about the boy? He doesn't need to see this."

Between screams his mother would cry and cover her head to protect herself from the falling glass. She'd been drinking again. "You understand me, Ewing?"

"Understand? Understand what, Claire?" his father asked, throwing another glass into the wall. "I-"

Smash.

"Under-"

Smash.

"stand."

Mason bolted across the kitchen to wrap his arms around her but was greeted instead by the backside of his mother's knuckles. Mason was sent flying into the nearby garbage can. "Get out of here!"

"Goddamn't, woman. Keep your hands off him. Boy, go to your room."

Mason collected himself and walked back towards his mother. He was crying now. He held out his arms to hold her and again was sent plowing into the wall. "Leave, Mason!" she yelled.

Mason hesitated. He wanted to help her. He wanted the fighting to stop.

"Get out of here, boy!" his father screamed.

Mason struggled to his feet and quickly left the kitchen. As the fighting continued, Mason went to his room and threw himself on his bed, covering his ears and eyes with his pillow. Each time he removed it from his head, he'd hear the sound of glass breaking or someone screaming at the top of their lungs.

After a while Mason spun his legs out of bed and walked the length of the hallway back towards the kitchen.

"I don't care about either of you," his mother yelled. Her words jumbled into a spitting mess.

"You don't? You don't," yelled his father. A powerful punch dropped her to the floor. Mason had never seen him hit her before. She scrambled as he kicked her in her side. "You don't?"

Mason ran towards her. "Mommy!"

Mason was sent tumbling to the floor, this time by his father's hand. His mother rose to her feet and grabbed a knife from the kitchen counter. "Enough!" she yelled.

"What you gonna to do with that?" his father asked nervously. "Put it down."

She shook her head. Her eyes were wild and she panted and heaved to catch her breath.

"There's no need for that, Claire. Put it down."

She refused to drop the weapon and started moving towards him.

"Put it down!" As he reached out to grab her, she swung hard cutting deeply into his arm.

Mason held his breath, his eyes wide with horror.

As she swung wildly again, his father fell backwards bringing the kitchen table down upon him. Overwhelmed with rage, she leapt onto him and lunged the blade deep into his chest again and again.

Although his body stopped moving after six or seven jabs, she continued to riddle him with wounds until she was too exhausted to lift the knife. She slid off his body and leaned heavily against the counter. Her blouse and pants were drenched with blood, and after smearing a streak of red across her face, she dropped the knife to the floor and began to cry. "Go to your room, Mason. Just go to your room."

Mason crawled from beneath the ledge and left the kitchen. Within minutes there was a knock at his bedroom door. Lieutenant Silverman. The next thing he knew he was in the back of an Oldsmobile heading to a hospital where he'd stay the night. From there he stayed at the county's child services center.

"Mason," said a large black woman, kneeling to better connect with him. "Your mother was committed to a state mental institution. Do you know what that means?"

Mason shook his head. It sounded bad.

Years later he learned that three weeks after the murder, his mother committed suicide by hanging herself in her cell. The state eventually awarded his custody to his grandfather. And Mason had a difficult time adjusting to life on the reservation. Not only was he plagued by horrible flashbacks, but the isolated life on the reservation allowed him few outlets to subdue his frustrations. With the help of his grandfather's ceremonies, hypnotic rituals, and religious teachings over the next six years, however, those memories were slowly put to rest.

"It's important to have someone like that in your life. Someone to guide and protect you," said Jordan.

"I'd be lost without him."

BOOM. FLASH.

The vision came strongly throwing Mason off balance. In a matter of seconds the faint image of a female entered his mind. Mason struggled to hold the picture together, but her features were silhouetted against a gray background making her difficult to identify. Mason grabbed his forehead and shut his eyes. The visions were growing in strength.

BOOM.

"Mason, are you okay?" Jordan reached out across the table and touched his hand. Mason jerked back and the vision left. The pain was instantly gone.

"I'm fine. I'm- I'm all right. I get headaches. I'm sorry."

"Are you sure you're okay? I can give you a ride. It's no-"

"I'm okay. Are you ready to go?"

From the restaurant, Mason walked Jordan to her car parked just across the street. Outside, Portland's bright city lights gave the overcast sky a pale orange glow. The Oregon air was cool and misty and the streets puddled in miniature lagoons. He stood close to the car while Jordan fumbled to find the right key.

"Are you sure you're all right?" she asked again, stepping inside as Mason held the door.

"Yes. I'll see Hawthorn tomorrow." He stood there in the light drizzle until Jordan had pulled away from the curb and turned around the corner. Something was changing inside him. He was at the water's edge. He didn't understand it, but he was getting closer to seeing his own reflection. Closer to finding the truth.

REVELATION

CHAPTER FOURTEEN

The morning sun had yet to peek its eye above the horizon when Hawthorn arrived at the Center's back gates. Howard, whose shift began at five, had no idea what was in the sealed manila envelope but appeared surprised to see Hawthorn at such an early hour.

"First one here, last one to leave," joked Hawthorn. Howard laughed, handed him the envelope, and waved him through. With his car nestled between the white lines of a nearby parking space, Hawthorn tossed the report into a leather bag along with the rest of his daily materials.

For the first two or three hours of the morning, Hawthorn saw various patients, making sure each routine check was thorough and precise. When he finished, he returned to an empty physician's lounge where he opened his locker and withdrew the bag. It was time to see what Williams' team had to say about Mason's patients.

Hawthorn entered one of the men's stalls in the adjacent restroom. The room, although designed like any other public restroom, was seldom visited by more than one physician at a time and figured to be the best place for a secret examination. He looked up at the ceiling. The floor. Williams had cameras all around the Center but it was difficult to imagine him putting one on each individual bathroom stall. Then again, it was Williams.

Hawthorn placed the bag gently on the ground and took a not-so-comfortable seat on the top portion of the toilet. As Nancy promised, the package was safety sealed. He opened it and withdrew a nicely bound, blue and white report.

The file was a summary of the police and internal security findings. Fifteen pages in length. Scanning the page, Hawthorn flew past the officers' names, time of inspection, and method of evidence collection. Eight pages later he arrived at the summary. There had been no evidence of forced entry, no apparent wounds to the young female, no indication of bodily molestation, and no evidence of chemical tampering.

However, there was one thing that stood out. Although there'd been no unusual fingerprints found at the scene, there were traces of vinyl. According to an article that Hawthorn had recently encountered, latex gloves could often cause allergic reactions in some individuals. One of the only ways to avoid this problem was to order special gloves made of vinyl. He couldn't recall the exact numbers but somewhere around three percent of the country's physicians used these gloves.

Hawthorn slipped the report back into the envelope and exited the stall. He figured he'd make a short walk down to purchasing on the first floor to see who in the Center used those types of gloves. He had a good friend there, one that could probably get him the information.

Hawthorn moved briskly down the hallway, swinging from side to side to avoid the other nurses, doctors, and patients zipping from one room to another. Several small children ran playfully through the halls as their mothers called out after them.

"Dr. Hawthorn," shouted a nurse, toiling over some charts. "Could you please take a look at this?"

"Sure. What is it?"

"Dr. Briggs isn't too clear here. I was hoping you could tell me the proper strength." She was referring to the number of milligrams of an antibiotic she was supposed to give the patient.

Hawthorn rested the bag next to his ankles and took the clipboard from her hands. After skimming the patient report, he withdrew a pen from his pocket and scribbled something on the top sheet.

"Looks like five hundred-"

One of the young children ran rapidly past Hawthorn's legs, kicking the bag down the hall. The contents scattered across the floor including the envelope, which slid for twenty feet, stopping at the foot of Dr. Williams himself.

Hawthorn froze.

Williams picked up the package and gave Hawthorn a deadly stare. He held the envelope in both hands, turning it over and over. Williams pried his fingers through the ripped opening, took hold of the document, and angrily approached as the nurse gathered the spilled papers from the polished tile.

"Dr. Hawthorn. What are you doing on this floor with that bag?"

"I'm sorry, Dr. Williams," Hawthorn stammered. "I was putting it away."

Williams withdrew his hand and pointed down the hallway. "But your locker is in the other direction, doctor." His fingers slipped back inside the envelope.

"Yes, sir. I know. I was helping this, uh, this young lady with some charts." The nurse stood nearby but said nothing.

Williams looked him over through half-slanted eyes. "Don't let me catch you on this floor with that again. This is a professional institution. Do you understand, Dr. Hawthorn? You know where the exits are."

"Of course, sir."

"Of course you do." He withdrew his fingers from the report and handed over the envelope. "You're being watched Dr. Hawthorn. Always being watched."

Hawthorn finished helping the nurse, and when Williams was far enough out of sight, he returned to the lounge where he locked up his bag and the report.

*　　*　　*　　*　　*　　*　　*　　*

"Hawthorn, buddy," said a surprised Gary Liotta. He'd been in locked in the basement's purchasing department with five other ten-key monkeys for nearly four years and shared their desperation for any human interaction.

"Miracle you're down here, huh?" Liotta spoke through a small sliding window on the wall to those who dared to start a conversation. His sleeves were rolled and hugged his shoulders, his shirt buttoned only halfway. "Like pulling teeth to get you guys to the dungeon. What can I do for ya?"

Although the room behind Gary appeared empty, Hawthorn could take no chances. He lowered his voice. "I need a quiet favor, Gary."

"Whoa, whoa, whoa there, buddy. Not your type. Not that I got anything against that sort of thing. Just ain't my cup of tea. Know what I mean?"

"This is serious. Listen to me." Gary's smile turned upside down. He now sensed the urgency in Hawthorn's voice. "I need to know who in the center uses Type II gloves."

"Vinyl?"

"Yeah."

"What for?"

"I just need the information, Gary. It's pretty damn important."

"Frickin A, buddy."

"And confidential."

"How confidential?"

"Very."

"Could I get fired for it?"

"Most likely, yes."

"I see." Gary rolled back from the counter in an old swivel chair, thinking. "Screw it. When the cat's away, the mice will play."

Gary waved him over to a large door that he electronically opened from his seated position. His office was a third world trash dump with paper stacks a mile high and a hospital form for every human on earth. Hawthorn stood nervously behind as Gary sped through a couple of menus on the screen of his computer. Using all six years of his community college education, he located the database that told him which products were delivered to which locations in the Center.

"Type I?" he asked again, his gold bracelets jingling as he punched the individual keys.

"No. Type II. Vinyl."

Gary hit a couple of buttons and the screen popped into a menu with a personnel listing for the past month regarding Type II vinyl gloves. "Here's your list."

Hawthorn moved in close, touching the top of the screen with his finger and slowly sliding it down. Mason had ordered Type II gloves twice in the last month. So had Williams. Moving further down the list he noticed that three nurses, Dr. Briggs, Dr. Rector and two other physicians were also frequent users.

"This what you wanted?"

Hawthorn felt his stomach sink. He was hoping Mason wouldn't have been on the list. On the other hand, Mason's glove prints should have been expected at the scene; he was her doctor. Without fingerprints, though, there was no other way to tell who else could have been there.

"Let me make sure I got this right," Hawthorn said. "Each of these people are allergic to latex gloves."

"Most likely. Latex is the sole source here. We got everyone's medical history in here somewhere. If I had clearance, I could tell you what you're allergic to."

"Who's got clearance?"

"Who do you think? Williams. Period. Don't get me started."

"Great. I think that'll do it."

"You sure you don't want to tell me what's going on?"

Hawthorn was already moving through the door.

"You don't want to know, Gary. I owe you one, buddy."

*   *   *   *   *   *   *   *

Shortly after his visit to the purchasing department, Hawthorn returned to the nurses' station to fill out the last details from a patient's report. He was already three reports behind. Williams would kill him if he found out.

Mason suddenly appeared at the end of the hallway. Between his busy rounds that morning, Hawthorn had tried to find Mason to question him on a number of topics. This time, however, Mason kept his distance, leaning heavily against the far end of the nurses' station. His skin bore a pale tint with tawny circles carrying blood shot eyes.

"Can you tell me where Mr. Johnson's been moved, please?" Mason asked.

A hefty nurse with a pencil lodged between her temple and ear answered from behind the counter. "313."

"Bolley Johnson's been moved?" Hawthorn interrupted. "Whose orders?"

"Family."

"Does William's know?"

"Yes. He's expecting Dr. Shane, here, at three this afternoon."

Mason hung his head and lethargically pulled his folders off the counter.

"One more thing, Dr. Shane," she added. "Briggs asked if you would check on one of his patients. He's thinking about transferring her to intensive care."

"Are you serious?" Mason asked.

"I know. I know," she said, waving him off. "It's Mrs. Rose in 390. Says her blood chem is way off."

"Just what I need," Mason answered.

Hawthorn hurriedly finished his report and joined Mason on his way to room 390. Mason hated Briggs. He had a nasty habit of transferring the care of his patients to the other physicians when the going got tough.

"Hey, you okay? You don't look so hot." Hawthorn moved quickly alongside Mason as he took long, marching strides. Mason said nothing. His face was tensed with apprehension. "Mason, I know now might not be a good time but I've got some important things to ask you."

"What?"

Both men moved to the side of the hall to avoid an oncoming patient in a mobile cart. Hawthorn faked a smile to the accompanying physician and politely nodded his head. Mason was not slowing down.

"Williams offered you a fellowship."

"So what. I didn't take it."

They were almost there. Three-ninety was just ahead. "A million dollars is a lot of money, Mason."

"Million?" Mason laughed. He stopped just outside the room. "If this has anything to do with this center, I don't really give a shit. Now, if you'll excuse me, I have a patient to see."

Hawthorn followed Mason quietly into the darkened room as the whisping sounds of a respirator filled the deadness of the air. To their surprise, Dr. Xiao sat quietly beside the elderly woman looking over some of her charts.

Xiao looked up at Mason, over to Hawthorn, and then returned indifferently to the papers in his hand. Between the men lay Mrs. Rose, an eighty-five year old great grandmother rendered helpless by old age. Her room was plain and cold. A couple of bouquets and a half dozen cards occupied the window sill but the rest of the room was bare and she alone.

From the side of her bed rose a giant tube that forced its way into her mouth, running to the back of her throat. Behind her was an army of electronic devices whose wires criss-crossed the floor like a deliberate booby trap. According to the charts, she'd been unconscious for nearly six days after taking some medication at home. Apparently her immune system was not able to offset the drug's side effects.

"What are you doing here?" Hawthorn whispered abruptly.

Xiao looked up from the chart and spoke at a normal tone. "Dr. Hawthorn, how happy I am that you could join us. I'm afraid this one's trying to cheat death." He handed his clipboard across the bed. "Look at her liver function, Mason. It could be a new record for poisoned blood."

Mason glanced over the figures and then handed the board to Hawthorn. Xiao was right. The numbers told the story. Everything about them pointed to damaged blood chemistry.

"Yes." Xiao was taking a degree of pleasure as he watched Mason gaze blankly at the woman's wrinkled face. "It's amazing she's still alive." He rolled the chair forward and leaned over the side railings on the bed. "Good morning, Mrs. Rose. How are we feeling today?"

"Knock it off, Xiao. You know she can't hear you." Hawthorn looked to Mason for input but he was lost in a paralyzed stare.

"Mrs. Rose, I'm afraid Dr. Shane here thinks you ought to be dead. What do you have to say about that?" He put his ear to her mouth. "Uh-huh. Yes. Dr. Shane is giving up on you."

"That's enough, Xiao," Hawthorn warned. "This isn't funny."

Xiao sat back in his chair. "I hate patients like this. Not alive, not dead. The best thing that could happen is for someone to give up hope and take her off these machines. But you can't do that, can you Mason? You're a doctor," he said sarcastically. "It's your job to save lives, not destroy them."

"I'm a researcher," Mason answered.

Hawthorn had heard enough. Mason was obviously not able to answer for himself. "How can you be so insensitive, Xiao? What would you do? Huh? What if it was your mother?"

"I'd do nothing. Absolutely nothing. For a patient like Mrs. Rose, that's the best thing you can do."

"Briggs wants to send her to IC," Mason commented.

Xiao smiled. "Briggs is an idiot. You know that as well as I do. How could her condition improve there? No, Mason. She has enough tubes in her here. A transfer would cost her family a fortune."

Hawthorn glanced again at Mason who appeared to give weight to Xiao's input. His eyes scanned over the elderly grandmother who appeared ghostly white in the dimly lit room. "You're right. Forget the transfer."

"Mason." Hawthorn said. "What the hell are you doing?"

"It's not easy to walk away from a patient who needs your help, is it?" asked Xiao. "Even if you are a 'researcher.'"

Mason was already moving through the door. "There's nothing I can do for her now. We both know it."

Hawthorn was stunned. He had no idea what to say. It was Mason's patient now and that meant Hawthorn had no control.

"I know there's nothing you can do," said Xiao. "That's the beauty of it."

CHAPTER FIFTEEN

Williams stood impatiently at the printer's side waiting for a document to come through the thin slot. He was in a horrible mood. Several of the Center's suppliers were experiencing strikes with their own workers which meant the delivery of gauze pads, bandages, and other dressings would be delayed another three days. The supply was already dwindling and according to Hector Denton, the inventory manager, the current levels would last maybe a week.

As he waited for the document to materialize, he noticed a small package tucked neatly beneath an antique desk. Curious, he left the printer and walked to the corner of the room, where he leaned over and examined the address. He lifted the box from the floor, shook it a couple of times, and set it down on a nearby countertop. The label read:

To:
Dr. Allen Williams
3805 Cellis Avenue
Portland, OR 62352

From:
Ladkan, Inc.

He hadn't signed for this. The fact that the package was sitting on his floor meant someone had been inside his office. Nancy always held the packages in the front room. He walked over to his desk and pushed the intercom button. A small red light in the lower corner of his phone flashed and after one ring Nancy answered.

"Yes, Dr. Williams."

"Nancy, I have a package in here from UPS that was delivered and signed for without my authorization. You know I don't allow delivery-"

"What package are you talking about, Dr. Williams?"

"This one's from Ladkan. UPS."

"I didn't sign for it. Either they just dropped it off, or... I don't know. Is there a date or time of delivery on the box?"

"I don't see one," he said, rotating the package in his hands. "Just the address."

"I could check with UPS. Would you like me to do that?"

"Just punch up their number. I'll handle this myself."

In a matter of seconds the phone was ringing. Williams continued to examine the exterior of the package. He knew what the contents were; he just wanted to know if anyone else did. All in all the wrapping looked unbothered.

"United Parcel Service. Can I help you?"

"Yes. I want some information regarding a package that was sent to me."

"The last name?"

"Well, I wasn't the one who signed for it."

"It's okay. I need the name of the addressee."

"Allen Williams. Dr. Allen Williams." In the background he could hear the attendant punching some buttons on his keyboard.

"3805 Cellis Avenue?"

"Yes."

"All right. It's all here. What can I help you with?"

"Well, you can start by telling me when, exactly, it was delivered."

The customer service rep punched a few more keys. "Looks like it was dropped off on the 15th at 3:18 in the afternoon."

He'd been at a Chamber meeting from two to four. "Don't you guys get a signature for the delivery?" "Yes sir." More buttons. "It was signed by Doctor... John... Hawthorn."

Williams' was shocked. This was a problem he didn't need. He hung up the phone and turned on his computer. After navigating his way through the introductory screens, he frantically searched through a list of files.

He quickly brought up the GENIOMICS file and his letter to Randy Edmonds regarding the potential dollar amount of Mason's fellowship filled the screen.

Williams turned off the computer and again forced Nancy into an intercom conversation. "I need you to e-mail Dr. Brenner and tell her that I'll be a little late to our public seminar this evening."

"Okay, Dr. Williams."

Williams hung up and then quickly punched up Edmond's direct number. This was a matter that couldn't wait for a private link up. Williams stood from his chair, looking sternly out through a set of large windows while the call clicked through.

*   *   *   *   *   *   *   *

In the other room, Nancy was having a hard time finding the e-mail password to Brenner's account. Each of the top administrators had special accounts to send each other executive memos in confidence. Beltman had suggested that the top brass receive special access accounts to ensure the safety and secrecy of their correspondence. She delicately pressed the intercom button and somehow was patched into Dr. Williams' phone call. Before she could speak, their conversation had commenced.

"What type of problem are you talking about, Allen?" Nancy could hear an immediate urgency in the other man's voice.

"There's another physician here who might have seen something about our offer."

"Might have?"

"Well, I'm not sure," said Williams. "He was in my office without my permission and might have seen a printout of the email I just sent to you."

Nancy wavered. This was none of her business. Just as she was about to hang up the phone she heard the other voice say, "We certainly can't take any chances. Get rid of him."

"Get rid of him?" barked Williams. "I can't just get rid of him. How in the hell am I going to do that? It's hard enough working with Dr. Shane. There is no way I can screw with two of these guys. Look, I've done my homework. I hear he's in a bit of a financial jam. Why don't we just offer him something? A fellowship."

"Look, Goddamn't. I'm running a very large company here, the consequences of whose actions either bring fortune or poverty to a lot of people. I'm not screwing around with some small time doctor who thinks he's going to be a cowboy on this. You offer him something small. If he takes it, fine. If not, I move on it. Now I've given you plenty of time here to do something."

*   *   *   *   *   *   *   *

Williams continued to stare nervously at the canopy of trees through his large, fifth story window. The sky appeared to darken on the horizon. "Yes, and everything's on schedule. The committee is having a meeting late tomorrow."

Williams turned around and slipped into his chair, playing with a silver pen on the top part of his desk. His eyes rolled over the paper holder, his computer keyboard, and finally to his phone where he saw the small flashing light. Nancy was listening and he knew it.

"Well, you tell me we've got someone else involved here," said Edmonds, "and I'm telling you we don't have time to be wasting on this. You take care of Shane. What's the other guy's name?"

"His name?"

"Yeah, give me his name. That's all I need."

As cruel as Williams' was, it was difficult for him to say the words. "John Hawthorn."

The little red light discontinued flashing. Nancy had hung up.

"What are you going to do?" Williams asked.

"Don't you worry. You better just do a little persuading of your own in the right area. You know what I mean? This is getting close. No screwing around. No one and I mean no one is gonna screw this up. Got me?"

"Of course, Randy. I'll call you after the meeting."

"Allen. You take care of business. We've got to clean this up before things get out of hand."

"I will. There's no way the board can overlook the loss of his second patient. I'm sure he'll be suspended."

*   *   *   *   *   *   *

Nancy had already picked up the phone and dialed Hawthorn's home. Her eyes bounced nervously from Williams' door to her intercom light.

"This is John Hawthorn. No one is here at the moment, so leave a message at the tone and I'll call you back as soon as I can."

Nancy hesitated. What could she say? She knew something was amiss, but what? She leaned in close to the phone and spoke in a deliberate, whispering voice.

"John, this is Nancy. Meet me here at the hospital at nine o'clock tonight. Something about Mason. And you."

*   *   *   *   *   *   *   *

Hundreds of miles to the north in Seattle, Randy Edmonds had already taken matters into his own hands. With his portable cell phone pressed to his ear, he reclined deep into a black leather sofa. His office was something out of a movie: black leather furniture, post-modern decor, white marble floors, and tall halogen lamps. The young executive was calling a number back in Portland. A number at the CME.

"Mr. Edmonds," a man answered. His voice was matter-of-fact.

"We've got a problem. His name's Hawthorn. John Hawthorn. You know him?"

"Of course. Another resident here. What can I help you with?"

Edmonds kicked one leg over the other and ran his fingers over the Italian leather in his shoes. "I told you I'd only call if the deal was at risk."

"Yes."

"Well, it may be time to elevate the game."

"What does he know?"

"At this point not much. But he could. We need to make sure he doesn't get close. Bug his house. Like Shane's. We need to watch who he talks to. What he does. He can't be allowed to interfere."

"And if he gets close?"

"Then he gets stopped."

"Stopped? I hope we're talking about something more than another hit and run. That wasn't pleasant."

"Whatever it takes," said Edmonds. "Wait for my word. This is just a heads up. In case we need to make a move."

"I trust you've conferred with Dr. Williams."

"No. And it needs to stay that way. Nothing's changed. If we have to do it again, he stays out of the loop. Just like last time. Let him run his center."

"Okay, Mr. Edmonds. He won't know a thing."

"We'll give Williams one or two more days to pull something off. Otherwise… you move on this Hawthorn guy. Same goes for Shane. Monitor every f'in move they make. There's more at stake here than anyone knows."

Edmonds hung up the phone and went back to his desk to check the latest stock price. He was pissed. No one was going to come between him and his fortune. No one.

CHAPTER SIXTEEN

Shortly after lunch, Mason was handed a note from Dr. Williams demanding he take the rest of the day off. Throughout the morning, Mason had fought through fever-like symptoms and new episodes of faintness and near collapse.

On his way home from the Center, Mason pulled into the asphalt lot of the Old County Library and went inside. He walked past several stacks of books on the second floor until he reached the collection on psychology. Mason hoped a return visit to the library would give him time to find the answers he desperately needed. He looked over the selection and withdrew a couple of texts.

Although the visions were dwindling in number, their intensity and pain were on the rise. His concern was not the pain, however, but the content. The meaning. None of the CME's neurologists offered answers. They performed many tests, but none presented resolution. It was his intention, as he settled into a sturdy wooden chair, to find the root cause of this madness; to once and for all understand the significance of each message.

For the next three hours, Mason read the scientific details of a medical journal, which recounted the case studies and causes for various neurological phenomenon. Although he suffered from many of the classic symptoms, he was unable to find anything where all of the characteristics he experienced were listed. After a while, he found it increasingly difficult to concentrate on the literature before him. He'd read three or four pages at a time, flip back and find that he could not remember a thing.

Removing a thin pair of glasses from his face, Mason stretched his long legs beneath the desk and leaned his head on the back of the chair. He stretched his arms and yawned. The ceilings were high, maybe twenty feet and adorned with original intricate carvings. He looked to the windows. The low afternoon sun beamed past the elongated rectangular glass giving the library a dusty, antiquated appearance. Mason breathed deeply and closed his eyes. He was exhausted. He hadn't slept much over the past few days.

BOOM. FLASH.

Mason was standing at the corner of an ancient Indian ruin. He could feel the soft dirt beneath his naked feet and although darkness surrounded him, he saw that the building was a single story dwelling located high atop a mesa in the desert flatland. From somewhere on the other side of the building, he could hear the heavy drumbeats and rhythmic chants of an Indian ceremony.

Buhm-ba-buhm-buhm. Buhm-ba-buhm-buhm.

The tips of his fingers slid curiously across the building's stones held firmly together by mud that had been baked by the sun for hundreds of years. He stopped at the corner and peered cautiously around its edge.

A shaman, wearing the ceremonial funeral dress, stood at the foot of a grave inside the circular burial pit. He wore a dark, rectangular mask with thin eye slits. Red streaks embellished the man's arms and chest in symbolic patterns. In one hand he held a long scepter at the top of which stood a black crow. At his side was a large, gray wolf that stared at Mason with unflinching eyes.

Although he could hear the drums beating loudly, Mason found himself alone with the strange Indian priest. The shaman was singing ceremoniously to a brilliant lightning storm looming on the distant horizon. When the chanting ceased, the sound of the pounding drums vanished.

The priest raised his scepter to the sky and slammed it into the earth, allowing the staff to stand on its own. The black crow then left its perch, flying high over Mason's head, and landed on the dwelling's roof. Either someone had died or someone was about to.

The priest motioned for him to walk forward, but Mason was paralyzed with fear. He gestured again but Mason refused to move. He wanted to run away. Again, the shaman demanded that Mason come forward.

This time Mason complied, passing first through the ancient burial ground and then to the base of the large grave. Across the open pit Mason could see four individual stones placed neatly side-by-side. A pile of fresh dirt lay next to the hole. The priest commanded him to look into the grave but Mason's eyes welled with tears. He couldn't do it. He didn't want to see. The shaman pointed angrily into the grave, insisting.

Reluctantly, Mason crept forward and looked over the edge.

BOOM.

Mason woke in a seated position, his head cocked toward the ceiling. He sat up and looked around, unsure of his surroundings. Nothing looked familiar. He stood and walked aimlessly down a long row of books. He felt as if he were floating. Mason turned a corner and headed down another long row of texts. This was the section of the library where the older books were kept.

Halfway down, Mason stopped and withdrew three texts, each from a section on Native American philosophy and religion. When he finished, Mason navigated back to his seat and began rifling aimlessly through their pages.

The first book had nothing to offer. His fingers danced through the pages without regard to their contents. The next was the same. Within seconds he'd combed it without luck. The third book wore a weathered blue cover that read, "Mi a ba djih" which meant "Sky People." The yellowish pages were stiffened by the passage of time and the threads on the binder unraveling at both ends. Halfway through, Mason stopped. Tucked neatly in the crease of the pages was a tightly folded, stale piece of lined paper. He carefully unfolded the note making sure not to damage the contents.

Directly before him appeared to be a scribbled map with barely-legible letters marking what he guessed were passageways. Beneath the map was a hand-written note, the words of which Mason could not immediately comprehend. His eyes scanned each line, not really reading them but rather looking for a key word. Finally, he stopped on the last line. The signature. Bearcloud.

Mason lifted the piece of paper from the book, his eyes transfixed upon the open page. On the right was an artistic rendition of an Indian man-spirit with long, dark-flowing hair. His face showed anger and his eyes were as black as night. He wore a vest of bones and held a long black scepter in his right hand that connected with the sky through a thick bolt of lightening. In the background was his animal spirit, an attacking Grizzly bear standing on its powerful hind legs, protecting the man.

On the left page were the title 'Bearcloud' and a small paragraph explaining the meaning and significance of the dark spirit. Mason stared blankly at the note and then at the picture in the book.

"The library will be closing in fifteen minutes," the overhead speakers declared.

Mason looked at his watch. It was 7:45. He was getting closer. He could taste meaning. Mason reached deep into his pocket and withdrew the small bottle of pills. Two more and he'd stop. Two more and perhaps he'd have the answer to his mental plight. He folded the note, dropped it in his pocket, and exited the building.

CHAPTER SEVENTEEN

Hawthorn returned home from a long day at the hospital at precisely eight thirty. Jordan had left him a note on the kitchen table explaining that she'd gone to get a cappuccino with a friend and would return around ten thirty.

After laying his jacket and leather bag neatly across a recliner in the living room, Hawthorn walked over to the breakfast bar where he saw the blinking red light on his answering machine. He shuffled through some mail. Nothing new. Bill. Junk. Collection agency. Bill. Lawyer. Late notice. Junk. He pressed play on the answering machine and made his way to the refrigerator looking for something to eat.

"Hi. Jordan? I hope this is the right number. It's Aunt Mickey. Just wanted to let you know that we're anxious to see you here in a couple of days. Give me a call around nine tomorrow morning and I'll give you directions."

Hawthorn withdrew a couple of jars and sat them neatly on the tile as he listened to the next message.

"Hi, John, it's Mom. Daddy's doing okay. I think he said your name today. Dr. Macon out today and… " He could tell she'd been crying. "And he said we should start considering the will. I didn't want to tell you but… anyway, don't worry about the money, John. Just do your best. We're always here for you. I love you."

Hawthorn felt an immense emptiness. They'd sacrificed everything for him. And now, with his father's condition slowly deteriorating, he was running out of time. He had to help Mason get back on track. His father's life depended on it.

"John, this is Nancy." Hawthorn froze. She was whispering. "Something about Mason. And you." He backed out of the refrigerator, slowly closing the door. Hawthorn pressed rewind and listened to it again. Her voice sounded urgent.

"John, this is Nancy. Meet me at the hospital at nine o'clock tonight. Something about Mason. And you."

Hawthorn picked up the phone and dialed Mason's number. It was the fifth time he'd tried to get hold of him that day, each time receiving no answer. If something had gone wrong at the hospital, he wanted to hear it straight from Mason's mouth. Hawthorn keyed in Mason's pager number and then headed out the door.

On his way to the hospital, Hawthorn passed briefly by Mason's home. His car was gone and neither the porch nor interior bulbs were alight. The day's newspaper was still wrapped in its rubber band and plastic protector at the base of the front door. Mason hadn't been home in a while.

Ten seconds in the main elevator and the doors slipped opened, revealing the lengthy hallway of administrative offices on the fifth floor. The overhead lights ran the length of the corridor and were off with the exception of a few emergency lights every twenty or thirty feet.

"Nancy?" Hawthorn jogged cautiously towards Williams' office. No one was working late. The entire floor was vacated. "Nancy."

Hawthorn pushed opened the door, slipped inside, and turned on the lights. Everything was gone. Nancy's empty oak desk sat neatly tucked in the corner of the vacant room. Every bit of paperwork, electrical wires, and wall decorations were gone. For a moment Hawthorn thought he was in the wrong area and then a nervous fear crept into him. He felt suddenly panicked.

Why would Nancy have been moved from Williams' office? Could this possibly be a joke? That's when he saw it. Beneath the vacant desk was a small piece of paper folded in half. Hawthorn glanced up to the corner of the ceiling. The camera was fixed on him, the small red light announcing the veiled party. Always being watched, Hawthorn, he thought.

Hawthorn positioned his back to the camera. Then he bent down to pick up the small note. Hawthorn glanced at the message, in Nancy's writing, as he slipped it in his shirt pocket: Geniomics. He'd seen them in the news almost everyday. Cure the common cold. Story of the year.

Hawthorn turned out the lights and made his way back to the elevator. Perhaps Cindy would know more. She usually worked late at night on her research projects and was known for being somewhat of a grapevine catchall for hospital information. Maybe she could tell him more about Geniomics.

Hawthorn exited quickly into the dimly lit foyer and up to the steel double doors that led to the mechanical workstations. He applied his clearance card to a proximity reader on the adjacent wall. The light remained red. He tried it again. Red. Again. Red.

Hawthorn examined the magnetic strip on the back of his access card. It looked okay. He wiped it clean with a small corner of his shirt and ran it through again. Red. Hawthorn pressed his face to one of the small windows on the door. From this distance, he couldn't tell whether Cindy was in the back. There were too many boxes and shelves in the way.

He tried his card again. Red. Jesus. How can something so simple be-

A light came on from inside the machinist area. Hawthorn pressed his face to the window and was about to knock when suddenly he pulled back. The light was

coming from Mason's research pod. From Hawthorn's vantage point, it was difficult to tell what Mason was doing. He pushed his face to the very corner of the window, trying to get the right angle but the pod's mini-blinds were half closed and further blocked Hawthorn's view.

He could hear the door slam shut in the other room. Hawthorn knocked heavily on the steel double doors. "Mason!" It was too late. The door to Mason's research pod had already shut. As the figure of a person passed through the light in the center of the soundproof pod, Hawthorn saw that the visitor was not Mason. The shadow cast on the blinds indicated that the person was wearing a full surgeons outfit complete with headdress, facemask, and gloves.

Hawthorn tried his magnetic card again. Red. Someone must have changed his security clearance. He looked back through the windows, further panicked. The person inside circled Mason's CoreTex machine two or three times, walked over to a counter where they had set aside a tool box of some sort and extracted a couple of devices.

Hawthorn pounded on the door with all of his might. "Hey!" The person bent at the waist and turned some kind of mechanism on the machine. Hawthorn spun around and pushed the button for the elevator. It was on the first floor. He slammed his fist on the closed elevator doors and ran back to the large double doors. The person was now extracting a component from the machine. Hawthorn banged angrily on the door but the intruder continued, unbothered and unaware.

Hawthorn retreated again to the elevator doors, rapidly pressing the button. At the very least, he could get downstairs to a phone and notify someone. The CME staffed foot security for the facility. They'd be the closest help. He stepped back and looked above the door. The elevator rested on the first floor and showed no signs of moving. He ran back to the large metal doors and peered helplessly into the mechanical room. The light in Mason's pod turned off and the door leading to the main workstation room swung open.

Hawthorn again banged on the door, surprising the intruder. "Hey!"

The man flinched and then sped towards the back portion of the room, heading for the seldom-used staircase.

Hawthorn frantically slashed his magnetic card through the narrow slip. Nothing. The elevator was now stuck at the third floor. Time was running out.

Bursting through the stairwell door, Hawthorn quickly descended the staircase. Within moments he reached the bottom floor and a hallway that would take him to the cafeteria. Hawthorn weaved and danced through the collection of empty tables and chairs, finally reaching a door that led to the main lobby. His body slammed into the door's handle, setting off the building's emergency alarm.

Hawthorn stumbled backwards and reversed direction towards the kitchen. There was a back door used for deliveries that should put him somewhere close to where the trespasser would emerge.

Ten seconds later, Hawthorn exploded through the unlocked door, exiting onto a seldom-used parking lot. The door slammed heavily behind him, muting the alarm and giving way to the low hum of passing cars on a distant roadway. Hawthorn stood there beneath a star-filled night, struggling to regain his breath and listening intensely for the noise of an opening or closing.

He moved cautiously around the corner of the brick building to find the back stairwell door thrown wide open. Hawthorn turned around and around but there was no one there. There were no voices, no roaring engine from a fleeing car, and no peddling footsteps of an unauthorized visitor. Disappointed, Hawthorn walked back around the

building where he was greeted face to face by a furious Dr.
Williams.

"Hawthorn. What the hell are you doing?"
Williams stood there with two of Beltman's security thugs
flanking each side. "What in God's name can possibly
explain this?"

"Dr. Williams," Hawthorn sputtered. "It's Mason's
pod. Someone broke-"

"The police are on their way, Dr. Hawthorn. But
what I asked is what are you doing here?"

"Someone asked me to me them here."

"Men, will you excuse me?" The two guards
promptly left his side and disappeared around the corner.
"Let's review the situation, shall we? You come here, at an
unusual hour for you I might add, Dr. Hawthorn. I know
this, you see, because I do your scheduling. Someone
breaks into Dr. Shane's research pod, we have alarms going
off, stairwell doors open… I think that's a little strange,
don't you?"

"Dr. Williams, I came here to meet Nancy. I went
up to her office and the entire place was cleared out. I went
down to R&D to ask Cindy if she knew where-"

"You're boring me, John."

"Someone altered my clearances," Hawthorn stated
angrily. "And someone broke into Dr. Shane's pod. I'm
sure if you check the hallway camera tapes-"

"Hallway cameras? Dr. Hawthorn, those are
dummy cameras. I thought you'd have known that. There
are no tapes. As I said, the proper authorities will be here
shortly. I'm sure they'll be quite interested in talking to
you. That's okay with you, is it not?"

"Of course." It was pointless to argue with him.

"And there is nothing for you hide?"

"What are you trying to say, Dr. Williams?"

"My point is, Dr. Hawthorn, don't bite the hand that
feeds you. Do *not* bite the hand that feeds you." With that,

Williams turned around and made his way to the front entrance.

"Where's Nancy?"

Dr. Williams hesitated. "Family emergency, Dr. Hawthorn. Said she won't be in for a while."

*   *   *   *   *   *   *   *

After speaking privately with the authorities, Dr. Williams sat alone in his office staring into a darkened windowpane. He turned on his computer, gained access to the security clearance menu, and brought up Hawthorn's file. The screen read:

DR. JOHN HAWTHORN   ACCESS: LEVEL I

Knocking Hawthorn down to L1 had worked well – nothing like containing a smart rat to a portion of the maze. Williams moved the cursor into the ACCESS field and changed the level from one back to two. There you go, Dr. Hawthorn, back with the rest of the clones. Before exiting he reviewed the authorizations for level three. Never can be too paranoid, he thought. His eyes danced over the listings. Satisfied that only he and Beltman had full admin and file access privileges, he saved the settings, changed the date of last access, and exited the program.

When he was finished, he sent Beltman an e-mail that said:

SEND ME THE TAPES. 4TH FLOOR.

*   *   *   *   *   *   *   *

For the next few hours Hawthorn sat with Police Chief O'Donnely answering more questions than he cared to. Three officers dusted the entire area for fingerprints while two others searched the back stairwell and parking lot for additional clues. The authorities tried to reach Mason at home but there was still no answer and, as usual, Mason failed to return his pages. They also confiscated Hawthorn's security clearance card and ran it through a few of the slips. Each time it successfully opened the door.

With his interrogation complete, Hawthorn went back up to the third floor to get a jacket from his locker. Afterwards, he traveled briskly down the empty corridor, past the nurses' stations and all of the patient rooms. It was late. To top it off, now it was time to face Jordan. She'd be angry that he hadn't called.

Just as he was about to press the button for the main elevator, the hollow sounds of approaching footsteps caused him to pause. They weren't the sounds of the usual soft-tread nurses' shoes. The closer they came, the more they sounded like dress shoes with hard leather soles knocking methodically against the cold hospital tile.

Seconds later, Hawthorn could hear two men's voices engaged in a whispering conversation. As the voices neared, Hawthorn panicked, stepping quickly inside a small janitorial closet. Williams would eat him alive if he found him on the third floor after the evening's theatrics. He slowly closed the door leaving open a small gap through which he could see.

"A job well done, Doctor." It was Williams.

"Easy as pie," replied the other man.

"Well, I've been here long enough. I don't suppose you'll be staying."

"No, no. I've had enough for one day."

"I agree," said Williams. "Enough for a week if you ask me."

Moments later the two men strolled past Hawthorn's sight giving away the identity of the second man. It was Briggs. Although he donned a t-shirt, his pants and shoes were covered in surgeon's scrubs. There was no reason Briggs should be there. Hawthorn knew he was involved in a research project on the fourth floor but he was never seen there past three in the afternoon. Furthermore, there were no patients on the third floor that weren't already covered by the staff on duty.

Hawthorn held his breath. The men were stalled somewhere to his left. It was difficult to make out exactly what was being said. The men took a few more steps. They were just outside his door.

"Sounds good," said Briggs. "I'm going to get changed and then I'm out of here."

"Have a good night. Good work today. I know it wasn't easy."

Hawthorn twisted his frame inside of the cramped closet. It sounded as if Williams was walking down a separate, adjoining hallway. From the fading clip-clop of his shoes, Hawthorn could tell that Briggs was moving down the hall towards the prep room where each physician would dress themselves in sterile scrubs.

Hawthorn quietly opened the door and stepped forward into the hallway. Briggs was nearing the end.

"Briggs," Hawthorn called out, his voice echoing through the hollow corridor. Briggs stopped. He looked surprised to see Hawthorn walking so quickly towards him. He put on his shallow smile and reversed direction to meet Hawthorn half way.

"John, what brings you-"

"What are you doing here, Briggs?"

"Checking on a patient. Why?"

Ever since the death of Mason's patients, Williams had made it clear that any physician wanting to visit a patient during the midnight hours was supposed to let him know at least a day in advance. It was done this way in order to provide the staff physicians with some feeling of security for their patients. Hawthorn had done it. Mason had done it. And if Briggs really was checking on a patient, it'd be reflected in Williams' schedule that was posted on the lounge wall.

"Is there a problem?" Briggs asked.

"What's with the scrubs?"

"I just bought these pants. I didn't want to get anything on them. Why are you asking such-"

"Have you been drinking, Briggs?" Hawthorn could smell the faint scent of whiskey on his breath.

"Wha- what?" He appeared offended Hawthorn would even ask such a question. "Give me a break, John."

Hawthorn stepped closer to him and spoke in a firm and direct tone of voice. "Have-you-been-drinking?"

"John, come on. I-"

"Answer the damn question," jolted Hawthorn. He was inches from Brigg's face. "I can smell it."

"I was doing some research." Briggs looked nervously down the empty hallway. Small beads of sweat now dotted his brow. He swallowed heavily and said, "It helps me stay calm."

Hawthorn spun him around and pushed him forcefully towards the doctor's lounge. There was a section on the schedule for research as well.

"What are you doing?" Briggs asked, struggling to free his arm. "Don't do anything you'll regret, John."

Hawthorn shoved him abruptly forward with a slight jab. "You better be on that schedule."

"I am. Chill out, John."

Hawthorn pushed him through the doors, escorting him to the schedule printout that was pinned to the wall above a lengthy blue couch.

"I'm on the schedule. Now let go of me."

Hawthorn perused the names and numbers until he had found the right date and time. Located eighth on the list was Dr. Kelvin Briggs, private research, 9:00 p.m. to 12:00 a.m.

"Where's your name," Briggs asked. "Huh? Where's your name, Hawthorn? I think you're the one that's screwed." Briggs stomped through the door, slamming it in Hawthorn's face.

STRATEGY

CHAPTER EIGHTEEN

"John?"

"What?" Hawthorn yelled with a mouth full of toothpaste. He spit again into the sink and rinsed the brush.

"Can you come here, please?" Jordan was calling from the bedroom, still dressed in the clothes she'd worn the day before. She must've been up for hours, Hawthorn surmised, and then finally had fallen asleep.

Hawthorn wiped his mouth with a nearby towel and walked back into the bedroom. He threw open the walk-in closet and shuffled some hangers back and forth. He could never find a decent tie. "What?"

"TransWorld called yesterday."

"Oh yeah?"

"Said they need some kind of good faith payment."

"And what did you tell them?"

"I said you'd call them as soon as- John, why won't you just accept a little help until you can get your feet beneath you?"

"Jordan," he said, backing his way out of the closet. "I don't want any help. I don't want anyone to carry me. I'll be fine. I'll have something lined up in a month or so and I'll be fine. Please. That's the last time I'm willing to talk about it. Drop it, will you?"

"Fine," she said. "I'm just trying to help. What time did you come in?"

"Can't tell ya," he answered, again rummaging through hangers in the closet. "Late."

"Why didn't you wake me?"

"Like I said, Jordan, it was late."

"Why didn't you sleep in the bed?"

Hawthorn backed out of the closet, again. "Just stop. Okay? I slept on the couch because you were already asleep and it was late. That's it. There's no more."

"John, I just want to know why you didn't call. You always call."

Hawthorn hung his head. He was such a jerk. Jesus, Hawthorn, mellow out. He walked around the edge of the bed and sat next to her. "I know. I'm sorry. I'm very stressed out right now."

"Your father?"

Hawthorn sighed. "I wish that were all."

The look in her eye told him that she understood he wasn't ready to talk. "Well, I waited up for you so that I could talk to you about something."

Hawthorn looked at the alarm clock on the dresser. He had to leave soon to make it to work on time. "Can we do it in three minutes?"

Jordan glanced at the clock. "No. It's okay. We'll do it later. But it's important, John." She straightened his tie and tucked it beneath his collar.

"I can't wait," he said. He kissed her gently on the forehead and then picked up his briefcase and left for another frantic day at the Center. After last night's antics, anything seemed possible.

*   *   *   *   *   *   *   *

As Hawthorn pulled slowly alongside Howard's gatehouse, he rolled down his window and stared up at the closed sliding window. Hawthorn squinted. It was impossible to see into the booth. He covered his eyes to protect them from the bright morning sun and contemplated knocking when the window gradually slid open.

"What are you doing in there, sleeping?" Hawthorn joked. "Vonnegut's a champ."

"I think you better take a look at this, Hawthorn."
Howard was pointing to a portable television in the corner of his booth.

Hawthorn peered into the small confines of the guardhouse. It was a news report on channel four. Katie Burns.

"When was this?" Hawthorn asked.

"I don't know. Must have been early this morning. I can't figure it out. We have specific orders not to let the media on the premises. Someone else must have let her in."

Katie Burns and her camera crew were just outside the CME's main entrance interviewing a young couple. Her face filled Howard's tiny screen. "Although the center's administration has yet to issue a public statement regarding Dr. Mason Shane's recent medical performance, it does appear that several of the hospital's clients are taking matters seriously. This couple has requested moving their young child out of the center's care and into an entirely separate hospital. Is that right, sir?"

A man with droopy eyes and a thin mustache stepped into the mike, eclipsing the main entrance from the camera's view. "Yes. We realize the hospital is taking proactive steps, but we don't want to take chances with our baby. Who does?"

Burns pushed the microphone towards the young mother. "And I'm sure you agree."

"Of course. Until they straighten things out, there's no way I want my daughter here."

Burns turned back towards the camera as it tightened in on her face. "As you can see, there appears to be a high level of concern among many of the center's patients. As I reported earlier, Dr. Mason Shane is under a preliminary internal investigation by the hospital administration, although at this time we are unaware exactly what that may constitute."

Burns held a hand to her ear as if she were receiving a message. "Okay... okay...I've... I've just received a report that..."

Hawthorn could see the hospital doors open as Mason moved solemnly down the long concrete walkway.

"Oh, Jeez," said Hawthorn in near disbelief.

"Not good," Howard agreed.

Burns rammed the microphone from her mouth to his. "Dr. Shane. One question. Dr. Shane."

Mason stumbled backwards. He was clearly off guard having an aggressive reporter and two cameramen ambushing him like a pack of game hunters. To make matters worse, he looked terrible. Hawthorn knew he hadn't been feeling well, but with two nights of no sleep, he appeared completely unkempt, almost wild. And now in front of the entire community.

"Dr. Shane. Can you confirm reports that you are under investigation for the deaths of two patients?"

Mason offered her a confused stare and continued walking away from the building.

"Dr. Shane," she said sliding across his body so the camera could get both people into frame. "Two of your patients in a month have died. Is there a conclusive reason? How do you explain this?"

Howard crossed his arms and stared at the screen. "I'd say your friend is in a lot of trouble."

Hawthorn stepped back from the monitor. He wanted to punch the wall. Who could he talk to? Who could he trust? Brenner. Perhaps she would have some answers. "Did you notify Dr. Williams?"

"He knows," answered Howard.

"What do you mean he knows?"

"Look." Howard pointed to the tiny television. Mason had moved away from the lobby while Burns paused outside the main entrance for a final recap. Thanks to the camera's wide angle, the silhouette of a man was visible in the fifth floor windows of Dr. Williams' office. The curtains were pulled to the side. "Yeah, I'd say he's aware."

"I just can't understand this," said Hawthorn. Williams hated this reporter. She almost screwed up his career not too long ago. Dr. Williams would never have let this happen. Not in a million years. He may have a strong distaste for Mason but why would he bring negative attention to his own center? He said good-bye to Howard and headed for the hospital's main entrance.

According to Williams' master schedule, Brenner was supposed to be in her office early in the day. She was the only administrator with whom Hawthorn could speak on even terms. She was the only one who had a positive history with Mason.

To his disappointment, however, Brenner's secretary would only say that she had stepped away for an unexpected meeting and would not return until late in the afternoon. She also surprised Hawthorn with a message that he and Mason were expected at an afternoon meeting in her office and that, most likely, Williams would be in attendance.

From Brenner's suite, Hawthorn traveled back down to the patients' floor where he stopped at a secluded pay phone. He reckoned Williams probably had some way of monitoring the hospital's phone calls and therefore considered this his safest bet.

The quarter clanked against the bottom of the empty machine as Hawthorn punched the seven-digit number. He twirled Nancy's note around and around in his fingers. *Geniomics.*

"DM Consulting." The voice was precise and business-like. It was his good pal, Doug McAfee. Network genius.

"Doug, this is John."

"My man," he replied happily. "What's up?"

"I need some information. On a very large corporation."

"Sure. Can you narrow it down a little?"

"Geniomics. A biotech. I need some insight. I really don't know... maybe what they're doing... like I said, I really don't know. I can get general info. You know, public stuff, but I need to know what is going on there. I need private information. Maybe their R&D. What's in their pipeline. Or new business ventures."

"Give me the name again."

"Geniomics."

"The cold drug?"

"Yeah. That's them."

"What's this for?"

"I can't really talk right now," Hawthorn said, keeping his voice to a quiet hum. His eyes bounced nervously between just about everything in the hallway. "It's very important, Doug."

"I see. I'm sure I can get something. I've got friends in some of the pharma research firms. And then there's black hat skills." He chuckled. "When do you need it?"

"Soon as possible."

"How soon?"

"Can you meet tonight? I can explain everything tonight. I really need someone to talk to."

"You're kidding, right? I'm a consultant for God's sakes. Remember? I get paid the big bucks for working long hours. Very, very long hours."

Hawthorn paused as a group of physicians passed on by. "This is important, Mac. Please. I know it's tough."

"What, like life and death?"

"Life and deaths. Seriously."

McAfee grew quiet. "Okay. Where?"

"Davenport Hotel." The Davenport was a beat-up hotel on the outskirts of town. Had to be safe.

"Davenport Hotel? John. What in the world are you up to?"

"Look, I just need your help. Trust me. You'll know everything tonight. Eight thirty. Okay?"

"What room?"

"Ask the front desk. It'll be under James Alton."

"James Alton," he repeated. "This better be good."

"And Doug?"

"Yep?"

"Not a word to Jordan. Or anyone else for that matter. No one can know any of this."

CHAPTER NINETEEN

Dr. Williams anchored the far end of a large conference table just as he had three days before. The same group of CME players were present at this second emergency meeting: Brenner, Susan Kinney from PR, security-wizard Karl Beltman, and the CME's top counsel, Dan Schwarz. Williams pouted in angry silence as he glared down upon a small stack of papers neatly organized before him. "Folks, we are about to have a major disaster on our hands. That damn Katie Burns was on this property... how, I have no idea. Perhaps Mr. Beltman can shed some light on-"

"Dr. Williams-"

"I'm not finished," he snapped. "Now. What I am looking for here, people, is an explanation. A bona fide explanation. I want to know what we are going to do about this television report. I want to know what we are going to do about Dr. Shane. And I want to know how in the hell Burns got on our property to air that report. Somebody better step up and give me the who, why, when, where, and how of the deal because I sure as hell know the 'what' part. Now who's going first?"

Susan Kinney nervously adjusted her glasses and said, "We've been bombarded all morning by the other channels asking for follow-ups. I called channel four and asked the producer to withhold the noon and evening editions until we've had a chance to make a statement. I know he canceled the noon report, although he was definitely doing us a favor. The evening newscast will replay the tape."

"What about our patients?" Williams asked. "Any more movement?"

Susan shuffled slightly in her chair. "Luckily, I don't think many of them saw it. It was broadcast around six thirty-five this morning. Most people who wanted to be moved have been taken care of. Just a couple. As long as it's not all over the news tonight, we should be okay."

"And the newspapers?"

"Everyone wants the exclusive. The <u>Oregonian</u> is planning to run the story tomorrow. I told them we'd have a statement shortly which bought a little time but…"

"Tell them a decision regarding Dr. Shane's future will be made public sometime in the next two days."

"They may not wait that long."

"How can we make a statement in two days?" interrupted Brenner. "We need more time than that. The lab needs more time. This is becoming unreasonable."

"Sarah, it is time to make a decision. I am *not* going to go over and over Mason's problems. You know them. We can ill afford to lose another patient. I don't care what the reasons are."

Brenner was disgusted. "You cannot implicate Dr. Shane of anything until we see some hard evidence. If this is your idea of justice, Dr. Williams-"

Williams stood angrily confronting her. "How dare you come in here and speak to me like I'm some child. I have been with this center for over thirty-five years. Thirty-five years. The changes I've made and the people I have employed have saved countless lives. People rely on this center to restore their health. To ease their pain. And I will not… *I-will-not* be responsible for another patient mysteriously dying under the roof of this building. Do you understand?"

Brenner fell quiet under Williams' furious glare as the other members of the team looked on, somewhat alarmed. The door opened and Dr. Clark entered, slowly taking a seat at the back of the room.

"Now," continued Williams in a more restrained tone, "I will give the investigative committee two more days to find any evidence it plans to gather either in favor or against Dr. Shane. But mark my words, a decision will be made. Am I clear?" Everyone shook their heads. "Am I clear, Dr. Brenner?"

"Yes."

"Two days. Next thing we have to discuss is how Burns got on site. Karl, this is your problem to explain."

Beltman sat at the opposite end of the table. His monotone disposition this day was supported a blue cardboard shirt and squarish, wire-rim glasses that carried a slight brown tint. Beltman's eyes danced over a security report. "I apologize, Allen, but I've been unable to pinpoint how she made it through. None of the perimeter sensors picked up intrusion. None of the guards reported any visitors and there were no signs of external power-"

"There's nothing on the cameras?" Dr. Clark asked from the corner of the room.

"Nothing, sir. Perhaps there was an internal power shortage, because we rewound the tapes and... poof... she was there."

Williams was shaking his head. He could see the uncertainty in Beltman's eyes. "Poof, Karl? Are you trying to tell me that an entire camera crew just popped out of thin air and did a report on our front door?"

"I'll check the tapes again, but I don't think-"

"I don't pay you to think, Karl. I pay you to prevent and react. To react to intruders that have entered these premises without authorization. What do we pay your people for? Did you give her permission to be there?"

"No sir."

"Well, that's good. Because neither did I. How could there be a power outage when we have redundant systems? Your data is bullshit, Karl. I need some answers. Not excuses. I've given you enough money to secure the

White House. I'll expect some worthwhile information from you in an hour. Next order of business."

Williams shuffled some papers and looked down the table to Dan Schwarz. "Is there anything on the young girl's family? I know her grandmother finally made it here."

Schwarz leaned back in his chair and casually swung one leg over the other. "As far as I know, she does not plan to take any action. If she doesn't contest the inconclusive result, I'd say we're in the clear. There is no other family and she certainly doesn't want any trouble. But..."

"But what?"

"Well, I hear the Center plans to conduct a second autopsy."

"And?"

"To be frank, Allen, if you open that young girl up again and find that Dr. Shane, or anybody for that matter, has tampered with her condition so as to induce death, the CME will be held liable."

"Liable? What the hell for? We didn't ask that son-of-a-bitch to kill her." Williams caught himself after receiving a hard glare from Brenner. "I mean, if an employee acts on his own free will, how can the CME be held responsible?"

"The problem is that the courts may see it that the hospital hasn't taken appropriate steps to rectify the situation."

"But we have a committee looking into it. What else can we do?"

"Yes," said Schwarz. "The problem is that you have continued to let Dr. Shane practice. You have begun an investigation but you have not discontinued his practice. Now, I realize that by terminating his employment we could come under-"

"That's because to this point, we have no evidence of any wrongdoing," interrupted Brenner. "If there would have been any evidence of foul play, Dr. Shane would have been suspended without delay. There are many cases where patients die for reasons that cannot be proven medically. We can't suspend every doctor, every time, just because an autopsy is returned inconclusive."

"I understand," said Schwarz. "My only concern is that one patient later the hospital finds a small piece of evidence suggesting foul play on the first two and then.... then we're talking problems. Major problems."

"So what do you suggest?" Williams asked.

"On one hand you could suspend Dr. Shane and open yourself up to a lawsuit for wrongful discharge. If you were later proven guilty of this offense, it would most certainly taint the center's reputation. After all, Mason is well known throughout the industry. Unless the investigative committee comes up with some sort of evidence, you would be firing him for 'no cause' which would be against the law. I must bring it to your attention that the center, and you in its leading position Dr. Williams, signed Dr. Shane to a three-year contract containing some hefty protection for him in the case of discharge. There must be cause. If it turned out that Dr. Shane's two inexplicable deaths were above the average that a reasonable doctor would encounter during a year, you would have substantial reason to suspend him. As it stands right now, two is not extraordinary and may not hold up in court as 'good cause.' Regardless, a second autopsy is not a good idea."

"And if he continues to practice?"

"On the other hand, if you allow him to stay and something later turns up that implicates Dr. Shane, I can assure you there will be heavy punitive losses in court for each count of negligence. Of course the best scenario is if Dr. Shane continues his practice and nothing else happens."

That did not please Williams. The CME, as it currently stood, had plenty of money to withstand lawsuits. The fact that Williams had an investigative committee in place as well as commissioned detectives writing special reports would most likely lower the punitive damages awarded to the plaintiff by the court. His concern was time. So far, Mason was making things very difficult. Nothing had worked. He refused to budge regardless of the amount of money offered to him and the committee had yet to move on the deaths of these two patients.

"Dr. Brenner," said Clark, resting his cane against the far wall. "I think this clearly underscores the need for your committee's report. If nothing is found, then so be it. Dr. Shane will continue. If something is found, we suspend him unconditionally and immediately negotiate a settlement out of court with each family in which foul play is evident. I think two days is a max."

"And if someone else is involved?" Brenner asked.

Williams turned his attention to Schwarz.

"Then the center should be fine," Schwarz answered. "If no one had prior knowledge, everyone will be fine. But like I said, if Dr. Shane is involved, I fear the court will believe this administration had the opportunity to put a stop to it and did not. Catch 22."

"That settles it," said Williams. "Ms. Kinney, take care of those reporters and issue that statement. Dr. Brenner, I believe you and I have an appointment with Dr. Shane in a half hour. And Karl, you better come up with something. I don't ever want this to happen again. That'll be all."

Once the other members had left the room, Williams again withdrew Mason's confidential medical file from his briefcase. After what he'd just heard, there was no telling how long the committee would take to reach a decision. Two days were worthless to him. There was simply no more time to wait. Williams flipped past

Mason's psychological history to a series of newspaper articles he'd saved from long ago.

For a brief moment, Williams looked over the papers, not really sure of what to do. He didn't want to ruin anyone's career, but he was being forced to make the big move. His future was at stake. Screw Shane. Williams placed the collection of articles inside a white envelope and sealed it shut. On one side of the unmarked package he wrote Mason's address. On the other, he wrote the words: 'Your secret is no more.'

CHAPTER TWENTY

Hawthorn waited restlessly in the hall across from Brenner's office, flipping through the latest copy of an orthopedic journal. Although he tried to read through the articles, he found himself looking nervously at the closed wooden door every ten or fifteen seconds. They were ten minutes late. What could they be talking about in there?

The door opened. "Please come in, John," said Brenner. Her voice was low and hushed with caution.

Dr. Williams was sitting casually on top of her desk with his right leg crossed comfortably over his left. Smiling, he pointed to a nearby chair, instructing Hawthorn to sit.

"Thank you for coming, Dr. Hawthorn. We have just a few questions for you and then you will be free to go."

Hawthorn nodded.

"I'm sure you're aware of the situation with Dr. Shane's patients, are you not?"

Hawthorn nodded. "Yes."

"And you were present at each autopsy?"

"I was."

"And you're also aware each case was deemed inconclusive?"

"Yes. Dr. Rector signed off on each report."

"And we had a little meeting ourselves last night, didn't we, Dr. Hawthorn?"

"I wouldn't call it a meeting."

"And it comes to my attention that you were later on the third floor, am I right?"

Hawthorn paused. "Yes. To retrieve something from my locker. My jacket and bag."

"But you were not authorized to be there. I mean you weren't officially on the schedule."

"Wait a minute, Dr. Williams, if you're trying to link my presence to-"

"I'm not linking anything, Dr. Hawthorn. I'm just trying to determine who was in the building late last night. People have been dying for no reason around here."

"Perhaps you should ask Briggs," blurted Hawthorn. He hated to say it. It went against all of his ethics to be a snitch, but in this case it was either Briggs or him.

Brenner appeared surprised to hear the name.

"This isn't about Briggs," said Williams, quickly switching the subject. "This is about you."

"Can I speak openly for one moment? Without being interrupted? Please?"

Williams nodded and said, "By all means, Dr. Hawthorn. Go right ahead."

"Someone was inside of Mason's pod."   "That's impossible," replied Williams. "He's the only one with a key. What were you doing on the fourth floor, John? I don't believe you were on the research schedule either."

Hawthorn was in a tough spot. He didn't want to bring Nancy's name into the conversation again. His instincts told him Williams was behind her disappearance. "I was going to meet with Cindy in the lab."

"Meet with Cindy? You could have easily checked the schedule to see that she wasn't working last night either. And then you claim that your security card didn't work?" Hawthorn had no reply. Williams stood from the desk and paced around Hawthorn's chair. "Let me just sum this up so that Dr. Brenner and I clearly understand the situation. You come here to meet Cindy, for a reason that is probably not important to me- research, I presume. You go to the fourth floor where you claim your security card isn't working but later we find nothing wrong with it."

"Dr. Will-"

"Let me finish. You claim that someone was in Mason's pod doing something to his device and then I find you next to an open back stairwell door that is only accessible from inside the research area. And you're out of breath. You reluctantly answer a few questions for the police-"

"I had no problem answering those questions."

"And then I hear you're back up on the third floor, without admin's permission. Is this story an accurate depiction of what took place?"

"I don't think-"

"I asked you a simple yes or no question, Dr. Hawthorn. Is that story an accurate depiction of what you were doing at the hospital last night?"

"Of course not."

"Then what about it is wrong? Were you not on the third floor?"

"Yes. I was but-"

"Did I not meet you outside?"

"Yes, but-"

"Did you slip your security card through research access?" Hawthorn didn't answer. "I know you did, see, because we have record of it. Yes, Dr. Hawthorn, I think it is a very accurate depiction of what went on last night. I can assure you that we will be in touch. There's nothing more. For now. You may go."

"Dr. Williams, this is absurd. Dr. Brenner, I-"

"That will be all, John," Williams sounded again.

Brenner hung her head, staring silently at the top of her desk as Hawthorn stood there, amazed, and then angrily exited the room. As the door shut behind him, Hawthorn saw Mason sitting in a chair across the hall. With his elbows resting wearily on the tops of his knees, Mason looked up and gave Hawthorn an expressionless glare.

"Where in the hell have you been?" Hawthorn whispered. "Christ, I've called you a thousand times, I've been by your house-" Mason dropped his head and looked at the floor's tile. "We have got to talk, Mason."

"I know."

Hawthorn could hear someone approaching Brenner's door from inside. "Be careful in there, Mason. Williams-"

"I could care less about him."

"Look, Mason, I can't help you if I can't find you."

"I've asked for your help, Hawthorn. If you want to help, then hook me up."

Hawthorn flinched. He could hear Brenner pause on the other side of the door as Williams doled out his final commands.

"Two o'clock," Mason said plainly, standing from the chair. "Café Express."

"What?"

Brenner cracked open the door and waited hesitantly at its edge. "Mason. Please come in."

"Two o'clock," he whispered as he brushed by.

*   *   *   *   *   *   *   *   *

"Dr. Shane, please sit down," said Williams, again pointing to the nearby seat. Mason ignored him. "Fine, Mason. Stand. Do you realize why you're here?"

"Of course."

"Good, then. We would like to discuss with you a patient by the name of..." Williams looked down at a small sheet of paper pretending not to know. "Miss Myra Floret."

"Yes. I've been expecting this."

"Great. Let me put this plainly to you. It's getting very difficult for us to dismiss these incidents as mere coincidence."

"So you accuse me of murder."

"Not at all, Mason," interrupted Brenner. "We're just trying to get to the bottom of this."

"I have nothing to hide, Dr. Williams. I am who I am. You're the one who told me doctors are not gods. People die for various reasons."

Williams nodded. "True. Yet in each of these cases the autopsies have been inconclusive. Doesn't that strike you as unusual? I mean, your last two cases. In a month."

"There are many unusual things in this world, Dr. Williams. As far as I know, she died from asphyxiation. Each case is well documented. If you're investigating me, go right ahead. You won't find a thing."

"Oh, won't we?" Williams asked, his face brimming with newfound interest. "Dr. Shane, this meeting is to inform you that, yes, as of today the Center is launching a full-scale investigation on the deaths of these two patients."

"That doesn't mean that you're responsible for them, Mason," explained Brenner, apologetically. "You are their doctor and we have the responsibility to look into these matters. Innocent until proven guilty applies."

"And we will expect your utmost cooperation," Williams added. "Anything short of that will be considered an act of incrimination. Do you have anything else to say, Dr. Shane?"

"No. Are you finished?"

Williams shrugged his shoulders and put on an egotistical smirk. Mason was getting the point. "Yes, Mason. I think so."

"Then I'd like to leave."

CHAPTER TWENTY-ONE

Edmonds stood alone at the windowpane of his twentieth story, high-tech office gazing anxiously across the Seattle skyline. Tiny raindrops speckled the window, distorting his view of the distant buildings. He looked up at the sky outside, spreading a formless blanket of gray. It'd been raining for nearly three straight days.

Edmonds winced, his hands gripping a waist-high railing that divided the massive panels of glass. What a grueling day. He let go and then gripped it again. Seemed like every VP had come in that morning to report a problem or ask for permission to breathe. It amazed him how few people were strong enough to make important decisions. Even high-paid execs were sheep waiting for slaughter. Edmonds yawned. Their hectic assault exhausted him to the point where he had his secretary clear his entire afternoon.

Out of the corner of his eye, he caught an incoming e-mail. The screen switched from its normal company icon to a three-dimensional silver cross. The message was enabling the decrypting function. He'd been waiting for Williams' report after his meeting with Mason. A few seconds later Williams' image appeared in the lower half of his monitor.

"Randy, good news. Things are looking much better. We'll have the final decision in two days."

Edmonds folded his arms as he waited for he image transmission to catch up with the voice signal. He looked into the camera, his eyebrows angling with concern. "Two days? You told me today. We're running out of time."

"I assure you. There is no way he makes it to the approval hearing on time. The pressure is taking its toll."

"And the committee?" Edmonds asked.

Williams' eyes bounced nervously from side to side as he considered his response. "It's public now. Two people? Trust me, Randy. They're ready to let him go. Two days, no more."

Edmonds bit down hard on his lip. "The hell with two days. This is getting too close, Allen."

"Wait. I received quite a surprise today. Neurology called. They found traces of Cyntocin in Dr. Shane's blood stream."

Edmonds' face suddenly lightened. "He's taking his own drug?"

"Shouldn't be long before we see an effect," Williams beamed. "No one knows his condition better than I."

"His condition?" Edmonds asked. He could hardly believe what he was hearing.

Williams nodded confidently. "Let's just say I've treated Dr. Shane before."

Edmonds was pissed. This exemplified the need to do something himself to get it done right. Williams was a fool. "Allen, let me put this to you in words you can understand. I am *not* betting my company on this physician's 'condition' or on the potential side effects of a speculative drug. You have a job to do. Screw two days. I want him gone and I want him gone now. You've been given your last warning. Do you understand?"

Williams' expression flipped nervously. "Of course."

"What about the rights issue?"

"Nothing to worry about, Randy. The center will have control of his research once he's terminated. He has no way of taking anything with him. Once he's gone, he's gone."

"Then finish him off. If that doesn't happen, we're in serious trouble."

"I understand. How are the tests? I hope there's been progress."

Edmonds leaned into his chair and kicked his feet up on the desk. "Still two to go. I've got people here twenty-four seven. L-3 tests are close. L-4 tests are still over spec."

"I'll cross my fingers."

"What about this Dr. Hawthorn?" Edmonds asked. He tossed his feet back to the ground and leaned forward as if he were suddenly curious again.

"Too scared to move. No more snooping for him."

"Good. You watch him, Allen. I'll be in touch. You can count on it." Edmonds exited the program and opened a thin sliding drawer beneath the center of his desk. On it was a myriad of buttons and sliding switches. The first three controlled each lamp in the room. There was one for a video projector, a stereo, and his intercom. He pushed the button labeled 'TV' and a large section of a far wall split slowly apart exposing a series of three four-foot screens.

He turned the middle screen to a "Moneyline" report on CNN. The PR team had secured the report featuring Geniomics at precisely 1:48 that afternoon.

Edmonds rose to the edge of his seat and rested his elbows firmly on the desk. The commercial ended and an attractive anchorwoman with penciled in eyebrows and high cheekbones began her report. Over her left shoulder was a box containing the Geniomics logo.

"We begin our broadcast this afternoon with a report on the rapidly growing pharmaceutical firm, Geniomics Incorporated. As you may recall from an earlier "Moneyline" report, Geniomics has consistently been one of the hottest performers this year, out earning the blue chips by nearly five to one. According to an inside source, an article is expected to be published tomorrow in the <u>Wall Street Journal</u> which claims the firm has allocated an extensive amount of capital to marketing and producing R2-X, a promising yet unproven drug."

Edmonds shifted in his seat, trying to gauge whether the broadcast was going to be positive or negative. Either way could mean massive fluctuations in the stock price. For him, each tick meant millions and a swarm of calls from his lead shareholders.

"You may recall that late last quarter a company spokesperson informed reporters that Geniomics R&D was finalizing the first ever cure for the common cold: R2-X. It was reported that only a small number of tests needed completion before gaining final FDA approval."

Edmonds winced. Eight years for God's sake. That's how long his most elite researchers had been working on closing out the cure for the common cold. There were no budgetary considerations. Ever. Whatever they wanted, they got.

The fact was that Geniomics was light years ahead of the competition in the ability to develop new drugs. "The Dell of Drug Discovery," Edmonds had once told Larry King. Edmonds was determined to leverage his visionary status in technology to dominate a more traditional industry. And he did, despite the shortsighted idiots at most analyst firms.

His plan was simple. While traditional pharmas laid fat with expensive Ph.D's squirting hundreds of concoctions into beakers in the lab, Geniomics was pioneering cutting-edge *in silico* drug discovery. One cheminformatic scientist, sitting at a simple PC terminal, now directed millions of three-dimensional models of drug-like molecules, slamming them against the modeled adenovirus target at a speed and cost previously unthinkable. If they docked with each other, he had a lead on a potential drug candidate.

Edmonds knew he'd have a cost and speed advantage. He also knew he'd lock out the competition on the back end with additional years of patent protection. To this degree, the company invested in millions of dollars of the latest compute hardware to speed the process. Geniomics even started a massive public grid computing service that would employ the idle processing power of millions of volunteers around the world to find cures for many non-commercial diseases. A generous move to win the public over.

Edmonds glanced at a stock certificate on his wall labeled '001'. He smiled. The roller coaster had been exhilarating getting here.

After several months of analysis, Edmonds' researchers eventually stumbled across a combination of chemicals that seemed to work on most test animals infected with the cold virus strain. Although their symptoms quickly disappeared, the researchers were appalled at the toxicity and rapid deterioration of the creatures' nervous system. Within seventy-two hours, the animals had collapsed and fallen into an irreversible coma.

Two and a half years later they had the second version of the formula that appeared to work well except for some respiratory problems found in a small percentage of human patients. Apparently their immune systems continued to treat the drug as a toxin.

Although most of the drug's formula consisted of synthetic chemicals and natural ingredients found throughout the world, there was still something missing. None of the necessary tests to gain FDA approval were passable. Late one night at the Geniomics R&D facility, a veteran researcher stumbled upon the missing catalyst: *Cyntocin* - an enzyme found only in the hearts of a rare South American frog.

Edmonds remembered well the pain of those days, the wounds fresh and the scars a mile deep. Geniomics had won approval to begin clinical trials and, after passing both Phase I and Phase II on a small number of patients, an FDA advisory group requested extended Phase III trials and final validation on several key issues. For the next twelve months his brilliant machine struggled to pass four separate tests. The first two had to do with the actual casing of the pill in which the drug would reside. These tests were easily passed. The third, L3, was a test to provide proof the drug worked as quickly as claimed. With mounds of inbound data delivered every hour, Geniomics' project managers were confident L3 would be passed at any moment. The fourth was a different story.

The inclusion of the Cyntocin enzyme in the R2-X formula complicated things considerably. As Mason's research would soon fully expose, there would be considerable side effects in using an enzyme-laden drug by itself, one of which included sporadic dementia. Although these post consumption, neuro-traumatic experiences were uncommon in limited trials performed for R2-X, the FDA would approve the cold-curing drug only if the reported side-effects occurred in less than one tenth of one percent of those who consumed the drug.

Geniomics researchers had conducted widespread clinical testing on people from across the globe and those results, at least those that remained, were just coming in. Currently they were running at slightly over three percent. Nowhere close.

An even larger problem, Edmonds knew, was that Dr. Shane's memo spoke of an incubation period for these side effects, meaning some patients would not experience psychosis for years at a time. Geniomics had been testing people for only the past two years and still were not able to hit the FDA's mark. If Mason was right, those numbers could blow through the roof.

Edmonds turned up the volume.

"It appears the market is interpreting Geniomics' road to approval as a positive sign as Geniomics' stock moved up three and a quarter by mid-day. Triton,

Geniomics' largest competitor, is expected to have its own version of R2-X soon but is not expected to make it in time for the FDA approval hearing. Their stock dipped six and three-eighths. In other news…"

Edmonds turned off the television, leaned back in his chair and spun around to view the cloud-filled sky. He had two risks. Triton was closing in on him and, although the market didn't know it, he did. To accelerate Geniomics' position as the industry leader, Edmonds had sold the board on a plan to invest heavily in the latest manufacturing equipment and technology infrastructure would be ready for operation the minute R2-X was approved. The investments were massive and spread across the globe.

The real challenge was that the frogs were non-migratory meaning they could only survive in their natural habitat. They could not be transported far nor could they be farmed in a synthetic environment. Cloning was attractive but years away. Many of these investments, therefore, were made right there in the jungles of South America. Irreversible. Edmonds was planning on a home run.

"We can't afford to share the enzyme with anyone," Edmonds said in a private conversation with Bill Simon, his co-founder and VP of Research and Development. "You know as well as I do that Shane will have a major corporation behind him once this passes and that'll kill us."

With such a large amount of capital riding on the success of R2-X, sharing the enzyme meant operating at half of Geniomics' plant capacity. Less product meant less profits and more time for a company like Triton to out-produce them in the market with more abundant ingredients. If things didn't go smoothly, Geniomics could easily collapse as an industry power.

There was a quick knock at Edmonds' door and Simon entered the office. Simon was six-four and built like a praying mantas with long over-sized arms, and slight curl at the shoulders. Unlike most researchers, he was socially capable, scientifically aggressive, and Edmond's only hope for a balanced conscience.

Edmonds spun around and closed the wall panels, concealing the three large screens. "What now?"

Simon had been in twice that morning complaining about an array of problems at the R&D facility. Apparently, the barrage of last minute results was overwhelming the scrambling R2-X staff.

"Nothing for once," he said, smiling. "We just cleared L3. One to go."

"You serious?"

"Yep. Jimmy ran the numbers six times today for confirmation. We're almost there."

"And the numbers?"

"On the network."

Edmonds' fingers danced across the keyboard until he found the destination directory where the results were stored. Simon waited patiently as Edmonds read over the columns of numbers on his screen. "This is really good. What about L-4?"

"Unfortunately, that's not so good. We're at three point seven percent, but Jimmy said he's got some new ideas."

"And our federal pals?"

"Nothing's changed. As far as they're concerned, the side effects are minor. But, I think eventually we're going to have to deal with them."

"No. Don't even say it. As long as we get those percentages down, we'll pass. Besides, we've got people working it twenty-four hours a day, right?"

"Yes, but-"

"But nothing. We'll get that percentage down below one tenth and then we're there. I don't care what happens, minor side-affects on one tenth of one percent of our users is not going to kill this deal."

"That's not what I'm worried about, Randy."

Edmonds dropped his pen and leaned back in his chair. He threw his hands on top of his head and rolled his eyes. "We've been talking about this for years, Bill. Again? It's why we started the company."

Simon glanced at the shut door and took a seat opposite Edmonds. "I know but I'm still worried about the timer."

"Why? It works."

"I know, Randy. That's the problem."

"It's brilliant, Bill. We're creating our own market. Demand that replenishes itself over and over and-"

"We're walking a thin line and I'm just not-"

"Why are you worried now? We're not going to engineer a disease unless we already have the cure. That's the model." This was nothing new to Edmonds. Simon had moments of weakness that only a solid pep talk from a co-founder could cure.

"We don't have the cure fully tested. If we release R2-X we'll suppress the cold but that time bomb will start altering the virus to form a new strain for a cure that's only half-baked."

"But we have three years till it releases. That's why we built the timer in the first place, right?"

Simon looked across the desk uneasily. "Yes."

"And R3-X is already being worked." Simon exhaled heavily and said nothing as he looked out the windows to the skyline. "Remember what we said years ago, Bill. Screw Mother Nature. We would never wait for her to put food on the table. Besides, the other guys have been doing this for years. We're just doing it faster. And smarter."

"I know," he said, standing from his chair. "What about the volunteers, though? If they knew…"

"They won't know," replied Edmonds. "No one can decipher the work and we're the only ones with the results. Besides we've done some great public work here."

"Randy, you told CNN and the rest of the world we were working on Malaria, not R2-X. They volunteered their machines for charity not for profit."

"And we gave the Malaria drug leads to public labs. Look, we needed to fill those systems between projects so we did. Big deal. We did the world a huge favor. It's over."

Simon glanced at the floor and then to Edmonds. "You committed?" Edmonds asked.

Simon didn't answer immediately. "Of course."

"Good. Don't worry. Once this launches, you'll have every resource known to man available for you to continue to press the envelope. We are there, my friend, and we're about to hit the very top. "

Simon raised his finger as if to make a point but was suddenly cut off by Edmonds who waved him out through the door. "Call you later," he mouthed, holding his phone to his chest. Once Simon was gone, he quickly dialed a number inside the FDA. Edmonds nervously tapped his finger against the desktop as his call transferred to its destination.

"Yes," answered an older man.

"Good news," Edmonds beamed. "We just passed level three."

"Glad to hear. And everything's documented?"

"Just looked over the numbers myself."

"Super. And the researcher?"

"Almost fixed. I've been assured-"

"Almost? I hope you realize what'll happen if it isn't."

"Of course I'm aware of that. I feel confident we'll be all right."

"I wouldn't worry about we, Randy. Everything must be documented. The ICC won't grant anything if the tests aren't verifiable."

Edmonds winced. The International Conservation Consortium was an international convention signed by every country, to protect and regulate the trade of endangered species. Without their acceptance, FDA approval was a distant dream. "We'll be ready."

"You don't have a choice."

"Well please remind your guys in DC which $250 million interest group got them appointed. We'll be ready. You just make sure your end executes."

His phone beeped and Edmonds switched lines. "Edmonds."

"Randy. This is Heathcrow." Dirk Heathcrow was Geniomics' Director of Public Affairs. "We've got a major problem."

"What is it?"

"It's Triton. They say they'll be ready to go on the 24th."

"What? How can they? They're three months behind."

"That's what we thought, too. They could be doing this to stop the slide on Wall Street, but if they're serious, and their tests are good..."

"Jesus," Edmonds cursed, his eyes bouncing across the room for something to smash.

"All I know is we better be ready to go with good data for the ICC. Without them, the Fed won't even consider us."

"Is the circle still tight?"

"Yes. But if the consortium says no..."

Edmonds grimaced and took a very deep breath. "We'll be there. One way or another, by God. We'll be there."

CHAPTER TWENTY-TWO

Café Express was an eclectic coffee house located in Portland's historic downtown area. The century-old building boasted high vaulted ceilings with heavy wooden beams stretching from wall to wall. Thirty glass-top tables were scattered across a dull wooden floor, and although most of the adjacent tables were empty at four o'clock in the afternoon, many of the cafe's employees continued to dart to and from a lengthy white counter, cleaning and preparing for the evening crowd. At this slow time of day most of the building's lights were turned off, the only illumination coming from the late afternoon sun that snuck its way past a thick band of clouds.

Hawthorn sat alone at a two-person table near the front window. He took a drink from his second cup of coffee, swirled the remaining contents, and finished it off. It was starting to drizzle outside. A couple of small children clung to their mother's leg across the street as she opened an umbrella over their heads. Mason was a no show.

A waiter stopped by with a fresh pot and offered Hawthorn a consoling look. He waived him off and then looked again through the now spotted window. He thought of his father and Mason's cure. He thought of Jordan, feeling ashamed that he'd put his job before her. It wasn't the first time. He thought of Williams and then his own career.

Then, out of nowhere, Mason came into view and was crossing the street. Though the mist hung like a curtain in the air, Mason carried no umbrella or jacket. His hair was flat and his face unshaven. He appeared to be holding something beneath his shirt.

Three seconds later, a set of bells hanging on the door jingled and Mason took a seat across from Hawthorn, dripping onto the table. Hawthorn pulled back, embarrassed, and looked around the cafe at the employees who stood watching.

"What is with you, Mason?" Hawthorn asked in a low voice. Mason was pulling a beat-up envelope from the inside of his jacket. "Jesus, look at you. What is going on?"

Mason placed the envelope on the table, disregarding Hawthorn's concern.

"Where have you been?" Hawthorn asked. "Have you even been home? What the hell is going on with you?"

"They're going to investigate me, John. Can you believe it? They're going to fire me."

"Mason, it's precautionary. I'm sure they have to."

"That's not important right now."

"I know you're upset about this, but-"

"Have you ever wondered why we're afraid of the dark?" Mason asked, his eyebrows flaring upwards.

Hawthorn's expression tensed. "Mason, I'm not up for one of your stupid games."

"Have you ever wondered why we're afraid of the dark?" Mason repeated. Hawthorn looked blankly across the table. "You see," Mason continued, "most people would argue it's merely an instinctive fear. We lose the benefit of one of our primary senses at night and are therefore more vulnerable to danger."

Mason leaned back in his chair, enjoying Hawthorn's confusion.

"Mason, I know you're having some problems right now but, please, I have no idea what you're talking about."

"We fear the dark, John, because it represents the unknown. And it is only when we are willing to face the unknown, and whatever danger or fate it holds for us, that you can achieve the highest of rewards. Knowledge;

illumination born out of darkness. I have something to show you."

Mason opened the damp envelope and withdrew a folded piece of paper, which he placed neatly on the table. He then unfolded the sheet, rotating it around to give Hawthorn a better view. It was a page torn from a book at the library. On it was an artist's rendition of an Indian spirit sketched in thin, pencil-like strokes. "Bearcloud," it said.

Hawthorn rolled his eyes and reluctantly studied the drawing. "What is it?"

"Not, what is it. Who is it. Look closely."

Hawthorn roamed the page glancing over the Indian man-spirit and the towering grizzly in the background. There was no caption. He looked vacantly at Mason and shrugged his shoulders.

"His name is Bearcloud."

Hawthorn examined the edges of the page realizing it had been torn from a larger book. "What are you doing with this, Mason?"

"Bearcloud was a powerful Indian spirit, Hawthorn."

"So what?"

"Don't you see, John? He and I are the same."

Hawthorn almost laughed out loud. This was more than he could handle. His patience was running thin. "Mason, I don't know how else to say this but you need to get some help. Listen to what you're saying. You're telling me- I-I don't even know what you're telling me. Possession?"

"Not possession, Hawthorn, reincarnation. Illumination born out of darkness."

"Come on, Mason!" Hawthorn said, raising his voice. An older couple eating in the far corner of the cafe looked towards them. Hawthorn collected himself and said, "Someone may be screwing with you at the hospital. I've been trying to tell you this for the past two days."

Mason had already leaned back into his chair, again dismissing Hawthorn's concern.

"Some strange things have been-"

"Who cares, John," Mason interrupted. "Who really cares? Maybe I am guilty. Maybe I killed that young girl."

Hawthorn looked nervously around the café. "Listen to me, Mason. None of this is your fault. There was someone in your pod. This may have something to do with your patients."

"Save your stories, John. I don't need you to rationalize anything I've done. I'm no longer interested in your help."

Disappointed, Hawthorn slumped against the wooden chair and stared hopelessly through the window. For the first time, Hawthorn realized he would have to accept his father's condition. He realized how much he'd counted on Mason's research, perhaps unrealistically so. Now he'd have to stand as the center peg of the family while his own father spiraled to a certain ending. "Think about your research for God's sake, Mason. You are *so* close. Think of all that can come from your project. My God, you're three days from helping a lot of people."

"Screw the research," Mason said indifferently. He took hold of the drawing with both hands. "This is much more important. A key to the past."

Hawthorn slammed his fist to the table. "Damn't, Mason, my father needs that treatment!"

Mason paused and looked at Hawthorn's teary eyes.

"I'm sorry," Hawthorn recanted. There was nowhere to go with it. "We'll talk to Brenner. I know she can help straighten this out."

For a moment, Mason showed signs of understanding, as if Hawthorn had broken through. Then, as easy as it had come, Mason's expression changed and he returned to his diluted stare. "It's too late for that. What's done is done," he said. "Let them try and find something."

"Please tell me this is a joke, Mason. I mean, please tell me this is some kind of joke."

"Not at all, John. I want you to meet me tomorrow at the Old Calvary cemetery. There's a very good reason why you should believe me."

Hawthorn threw an elbow onto the table and buried his forehead in the palm of his hand. "Why?"

"I have proof." Mason reached again into the weathered envelope and withdrew an old black and white photograph. He pushed it across the table and into Hawthorn's view. For a moment, the tenseness in Hawthorn's face vanished as his eyebrows lifted with curiosity. Directly before him lay a photo of an old gravesite. "This is who I used to be. My name was Shepard Boone."

CHAPTER TWENTY-THREE

It was wartime for Randy Edmonds and the Geniomics executive team. Triton's announcement the following morning would mean a halt to the recent increases in Geniomics stock price and possibly a heavy decline. Edmonds knew his major stockholders would be calling at the break of dawn to find out how serious his miscalculation had been. It was now an information game, each company issuing statements to the press hoping to influence the market's perception of what was about to occur.

Edmonds' office resembled a combat bunker: hundreds of pieces of paper strewn about the floor, vice presidents yapping on their cell phones while they paced around his office, and three large television screens glowing with the latest numbers from Wall Street.

"Wally," Edmonds yelled from across the room. Walter Crooks was Geniomics' VP of Finance and considered one of the best in the business. He'd been hired away from Triton three years before for an "extreme" salary.

Edmonds sat behind his desk glaring at his computer screen now tied real time to the NASDAQ ticker. "Where the hell are those numbers?" Crooks' team of bean counters was to deliver a slew of financial scenarios that would result from varying Triton announcements.

"Working on it," Crooks answered, his own ear taken up by a portable phone. "Within the hour."

"Tell 'em that's not good enough. I need those numbers now."

"Randy. Line four," shouted his executive assistant.

Edmonds picked up the phone at the edge of his desk. "Yeah."

"Randy. It's Ted." Ted Malley was Geniomics head of South American Operations. He was directly responsible for the new facility in Macapa, Brazil that was expected to begin production minutes after R2-X was approved by the ICC and FDA.

"Did you hear about Triton?" asked Edmonds.

"Just now. Pisses me off. Where are we?"

"Down three and a half."

"Crap. Think Triton's serious?"

"Hard to tell," Edmonds replied. "They won't return my calls."

"What about them?

"Up two and three-eighths."

"Bastards. And our tests?"

"We're at level four. Passed L3 early this morning."

"At least that's encouraging." There was a short silence on Malley's end. "Uh, Randy, we've got an additional problem."

"Christ. What now?"

"It's the government down here. They just sent a representative to my office. I guess we're not the only one who saw that report. They're worried about us defaulting on our payments for the lab and plant if Triton launches something anywhere near us. They're thinking about withholding our tax credits until we can show more-"

"They can't do that. We have an agreement with their Minister."

"Randy. These people don't give a rat's ass. When the shit hits the fan, they cover their butts any way they can."

"What do they want?"

"Who knows? They're worried like the rest of us. If that plant doesn't open in full force, two thousand potential jobs go down with it. They're worried."

"Is everything in place down there?"

"We'll be fully operational in three days. We've had some problems with a couple of the generators but for the most part, we're waiting on the go ahead from you guys."

"I'll take care of the Minister. You get those people ready to go. If Triton's serious, we'll have to move as quick as possible. I'm talking very large batches right off the bat. Our channels are spreading like wildflowers over here. If that thing has to stay open twenty-five hours a day, so be it."

"Okay, Randy. I'll wait for your call. Good luck."

"I don't need luck. I need my people to perform."

Edmonds hung up the phone, stood behind his desk, and called out to the others in the room. "All right, folks. Listen up. We've got some major problems on our hands. The Brazilian government is getting restless and our stock is dropping like a fat man off a diving board. Wally, those numbers?"

Crooks shook his head. "Any minute now."

"Okay. Two things. I want to know exactly what our bottom line is going to look like for the next five quarters if Triton makes the FDA's hearing and markets their clone anywhere within three months of us. Give me the return on sales, unit forecasts and margins. Take the numbers down to EBITDA and earnings per share. I want to know what this is going to look like to investors."

Crooks nodded and made another phone call.

"Camden." Ken Camden was the Geniomics Vice President of Marketing. He was dressed in a light blue shirt with his sleeves rolled up to his elbows and a cell phone pressed tightly against his ear. "I want to see some pricing and cost analysis done for the next five quarters assuming Triton is there in the market holding our hand. Find out which of our suppliers we can squeeze. We may be going to bed with them, but it doesn't mean we can't cheat."

Edmonds' phone rang. "Yeah."

"Randy. It's Simon. We're back up to three and a half percent on these damn tests. We thought we had it, but the samples were bad. I just thought you should know."

Edmonds crushed a paper coffee cup with his fist, startling the others in the room. "Well, when the hell do the next samples come in?"

"Tomorrow at eight."

"That's too late. We're getting killed out there."

"There's nothing else I can do. We've run through all the tests twice. We're not even close."

A courier entered the room with a few sheets of paper and delivered them to Crooks.

"How many more batches can we expect?"

"Three more. Two tomorrow. We'll certainly have something for the ICC."

"Jesus. That's not good enough. Hang on."

Geniomics' latest price was quickly approaching on the NASDAQ ticker. The market would close in fifteen minutes.

... GEA up 1 1/4 ... GEF down 2 1/8 ... GEJ up 3/8

All movement in the room suspended as each man's vision funneled towards the screen.

... GEN down 8 1/8 ...

Edmonds sank back into his chair.

"Randy. What is it? Randy?"

"I'm here. We're down 8 1/8."

"Oh, man."

Crooks was waving for Edmonds to get off the phone.

"Bill, I'll call you right back." Crooks placed the stack of papers in front of him. He looked worried.

Edmonds turned down the sound on all three screens. His eyes rolled slowly across the page moving up and down the columns of numbers. When he finished, he sat them down on his desk and looked helplessly up at Crooks. "Are these accurate?"

"I believe so. Yes."

Edmonds put his face between his hands and ran his fingers through his hair. Camden had stopped talking on his phone and waited patiently for Edmonds' reaction from across the room.

"Fine," Edmonds said calmly. He excused everyone else from his office and motioned for Camden and Crooks to follow him to a visiting area where two couches cornered a designer glass coffee table. The two vice presidents sat nervously side by side as Edmonds reached around a lamp next to his chair and picked up the phone. He punched a button tying him directly to Simon at the R&D facility.

"Bill, this is Randy again," he said. "We just received the latest financials and…" He looked to the other men who quietly awaited the verdict. "And I'm going to hold a press conference tomorrow announcing that Geniomics has passed all four of our final tests."

Camden fell back into the sofa's cushions while Crooks remained seated at the edge of the couch, staring down at the floor with an emotionless expression.

"Tomorrow?" Simon asked. "We'll just be getting the next batches."

"I know that, Bill," Edmonds replied. "But this company will go down in a hurry. Do you understand? We're down eight and an eighth right now and the market knows we're banking on approval and at least three months lead-time over Triton. If I don't give them something positive tomorrow, the livelihood of every Geniomics family will be in jeopardy."

"But it's only a swing in the stock price."

"It's much more than that. We've risked a lot here. More than you know."

"Randy, I understand the predicament."

Edmonds face tensed. "Bill, I know you don't understand the predicament. We have three more samples from which to draw less than one-tenth. We have three batches coming. That's it. Those groups are our last three chances. I'm going to explain to them that we passed L4. You'd have passed it anyway, right?"

"Randy-"

"Right?" Simon gave no answer. "Put it this way. I know you'll pass those tests. I am sure of that."

Simon remained quiet for a moment and then said, "Randy, please. We're at three and half right now and I just don't see how we can pass them. You have to be reasonable."

"They will *not* fail. Do we understand each other?"

Simon sighed and reluctantly said, "Yes, Randy. I understand."

"They'll be taken care of. Fill your top two people in on the details. And remind them they're under a full NDA. No whistle blowers, you understand me? I'll be happy to spend every last Geniomics dollar to punish them."

Edmonds hung up the phone and looked calmly at the other men across the room. Camden nervously rubbed his forehead with one hand while Crooks continued to gaze at the floor in silence. "You two may or may not agree with what is about to happen and you may or may not agree with things I've done in the past. But I need your support right this second. The one thing I've learned in this industry is that the future is purchased by the present. Sometimes you simply have to do whatever it takes to win. Bottom line."

"Randy," Camden implored. "Do you realize what you're doing?"

"Gentlemen, I refuse to punish this company for bravely taking strides in a direction where no company has ever been. If we pass the L-4 test, millions of people will benefit. If we fail, we always have the option not to market the drug. But I adamantly decline to let this company be driven into the ground without ever knowing whether we hold the key to suppressing the common cold. Or pneumonia. The potential to cure millions of people. I need your support. You have my word that I will do everything in my power to lower our L-4s within the first few days our product is out there."

"People will suffer," Camden stressed.

"Yes, a few will be pioneers. A few will suffer for the good of humanity. Everything possible will be done to alleviate that. But I'm making that announcement tomorrow. Do either of you have anything else to add?"

There was no reply from either man.

"Then that'll be all."

When the men had left his office, Edmonds made a private phone call to Portland. To the CME.

"Yes?"

"It's me, Randy. Time to make another move. Time to give the dogs a bone. I simply cannot wait for Williams' efforts."

"I trust this is the plan we've discussed."

"Yes," Edmonds answered. "There's another piece of the puzzle you should know. In a couple of days, we put in application for an ingredient critical to the success of R2-X. An application to the ICC. Dr. Shane cannot make it to that hearing. More specifically, his research."

"Elimination?"

"No. That would draw too much attention. Besides, it appears Dr. Shane is taking himself out of the picture."

"So what you need is…"

"The one I'm worried about is this Dr. Hawthorn character. He's taking a keen interest in late night excursions to the Center. Williams notified me that he might have some potentially damaging information. I can no longer afford to take any chances. Keep your eye on him."

"Yes, sir. And the dogs will have their bone."

CHAPTER TWENTY-FOUR

The Davenport Hotel was a single story, light blue building located at the outskirts of town, along a road that used to serve Portland as the main highway going to and from San Francisco. Before the newer Highway 5 was built, every traveler coming to Portland from Northern California would pass through, stopping to shop at nearby stores and eat at the now-extinct restaurants. The Davenport was perhaps the last visual reminder of the era's heyday, and although the newer system of freeways had long depleted the area's businesses, the hotel's owner had kept the dwelling open, splitting the business between less fortunate families who needed an inexpensive place to live and tourists who were obviously lost.

Hawthorn pulled back the curtains and peeked out through the narrow opening. He'd been waiting for what seemed like hours in the monotonous confines of room twenty-four. Across the roadway, he could see the skeletal framework of ghost-like buildings and vacant lots. The evening sky was cloudless and provided a violet backdrop for a large red and white neon sign that flashed "Davenport" at the edge of the entrance. There were five cars in the immediate lot, all of which had been there when Hawthorn first arrived.

For the most part, there was little movement outside Hawthorn's room. Occasionally he'd see a couple of children playing around a swing set in the middle of a lighted, grassy area near the pool. Every five minutes a doorway across the way, number three, would open as a fat man with stains on his belly yelled at the kids.

Hawthorn released the curtains and sat on the edge of the bed. McAfee should be there any moment. He threw a couple of limp pillows behind his head and kicked his feet up on the mattress. The bed gave off a cheap, plastic-crumpling sound. He hadn't felt this tired in years. Maybe he'd rest for a minute or two.

A car's engine turned off outside his window and Hawthorn spun out of bed. Through the narrow slit he could see a newer, burgundy Lincoln Town car located three spots down from his door. Whoever was driving was no longer in the vehicle. It wasn't McAfee. He drove a Mercedes.

Suddenly, Hawthorn heard footsteps just outside his door. He released the curtains and froze. The door handle wriggled back and forth.

Hawthorn glanced at the thin safety bar locking the door. It was barely fastened. He searched the backside for a peephole on the door but there wasn't one. If he crossed the window, a shadow would be cast on the pane.

Beep. Beep. Beep. Beep.

Hawthorn's cell phone rang loudly from across the room.

"John," sounded McAfee as he rapped on the door. Hawthorn calmed himself and opened it. "Sorry I'm late. Had to get a rental. Damn car broke down."

Hawthorn pulled him quickly inside and re-locked the door. "You scared the hell out of me."

"Nice location."

"There's a good reason for it."

For the next twenty minutes, Hawthorn told him everything. He began with a detailed account of the two autopsies, how Mason had done everything by the book and still there were no conclusions to be drawn. He then discussed Beltman's file and the traces of vinyl. Hawthorn told him how he'd gone to purchasing and who he'd found on the list.

Next, he recounted the letter he found in William's office regarding Mason and the dollar amount of the research opportunity. He told him of Nancy's disappearance and the small note left behind with the word "Geniomics." Then there was the perpetrator in Mason's pod, and lastly, Mason's problems. How it was almost impossible to speak with him.

McAfee sat opposite Hawthorn on one of the twin beds assimilating what he had heard. "Have you told Mason what you know?"

"I've tried. He isn't listening to anything."

"Sounds like someone's setting him up."

"I think so too, but-" Hawthorn hated to say it.

"But what?"

"Mason's starting to think he may be responsible."

"He doesn't know?" McAfee asked.

"He's having some serious problems right now. Depression, anxiety, blackouts... I just don't know. Hell, everything's wrong with him."

"And he is on the glove list," McAfee confirmed.

Hawthorn stood and paced back and forth in front of the television. "All these random events..."

"Do *you* think he did it?"

Hawthorn stopped pacing. "To tell you the truth, right now I really don't know. I can't picture him doing anything like that but... he's changing."

"Changing?"

"It's hard to define. Like a clock winding down. Each time I talk to him he makes less and less sense."

"I'm sure you've thought about going to the police."

"Of course. But what do I have to show? I certainly don't want to piss away my own career. And I have no proof of anything."

"What about this Dr. Brenner? You told me you could trust her."

"Yeah. She was at the meeting today, too. Didn't say a word. It's hard to know who I can trust right now. For all I know, she may be involved."

"I don't know," said McAfee, pensively shaking his head. "I still think there's more to it than that. Take a step back and try to look for any common thread that ties these events together. From what you've told me, there's some kind of link between Geniomics and Dr. Williams. You saw a letter from Williams to their CEO. And they offered Mason a ton of money."

"Uh-huh."

"There's one. Now, some strange things have been going on at the hospital, right?"

Hawthorn nodded.

"William's secretary disappears right before you're supposed to meet with her... you catch this Briggs guy talking and laughing with Williams right after you see someone messing with Mason's research... and then Williams makes it look like you might be the guilty party. I'd say he's definitely involved. And he's on to you. There's two. You put one and two together and I say you might find something."

"And where does Mason fit in?" Hawthorn asked. "I mean, how is that going to help me find out who's actually killing Mason's patients? Assuming he's not... you know."

"I don't know," said McAfee, all you can do is follow the link between Geniomics and Dr. Williams; why they want Mason out of the picture or on their payroll. If you don't find anything, then at least one possible avenue has been exhausted."

"And then what?" Hawthorn asked. He felt like a naïve child, completely unable to frame the problem.

"You said someone was tinkering with his machine right?"

"Yes."

"That tells me they may not like what he's working on."

"Or maybe they just don't like him," replied Hawthorn.

"True." McAfee reached into a briefcase and withdrew a collection of papers. "I got the info you requested on Geniomics."

He handed half of the stack to Hawthorn. "Geniomics is a young but very powerful pharmaceutical company with an extremely high potential for growth. They've been in the news quite a bit lately. Have you seen?"

Hawthorn nodded. They were practically in every newscast.

"Their stock price has been swinging in fairly wide fluctuations lately. Mostly down in the last couple of weeks. From what I gather, they anticipated beating their competition to the market by a couple of years. Evidently their competition, Triton, just announced today that they plan on hitting the market at close to the same time, so Geniomics' revenues will probably not be anywhere near what they were planning. Take a look at this." McAfee handed Hawthorn a copy of Geniomics' annual report.

As Hawthorn thumbed through the glossy manual, he could see evidence of McAfee's explanation. Apparently Geniomics was investing quite heavily into plant, property, and equipment. Their sales force had nearly quintupled. The report centered around R2-X and how it was destined to make Geniomics the world's premier pharmaceutical firm.

Once past the Director's note and financial statements, Hawthorn turned to a page listing the Board members and the companies they currently represented. The list was impressive. Executives from some Fortune 500 companies obviously had some stake in Geniomics' operation. The only one without a company was Sam A. Mullin. Everyone else was an American corporate hero.

Sam A. Mullin

He'd seen the name somewhere but couldn't place it. Nothing else really jumped at him, at least nothing that gave him a clue as to what else Geniomics could be doing. Hawthorn turned back to the listing of the members of the board. "I need you to check on a few of these names."

"Okay." McAfee scrambled for a pen. "What good is that going to do?"

"I have no idea. A couple of these names sound familiar. I can't remember where I've seen them."

"All right, but don't get your hopes up. Most of these people are public figures I would imagine: heads of major corporations, noted investors. I can do some prelim searching on the net, but I can take it a step further..."

"Further?"

"Let's just say I've got this buddy in DC who's great at this stuff. We may need to shoot him a couple of bucks, but he's good. He can get anything. I don't ask how he does it and, to tell you the truth, we probably don't want to know."

"Fine. Send me an email with a quote. Put him on Delvin Kants, Gerard Bishop, and Sam Mullin."

"What're we looking for exactly?" McAfee asked as he scribbled each name onto some complimentary paper.

"Good question. Personal history, education, employment, credit, investments, social circles, whatever you can get. Take a stab. Otherwise, I need time to think of what other direction we can take."

"All right, Hawthorn. I'll get back to you on this as soon as I can. This company's a powerhouse, though. They're liquid, profitable, and they're growing like mad."

Hawthorn shrugged his shoulders and shook his head. "You see? That's the thing. Mason's research has nothing to do with the common cold."

"Then I'd say you should try and find out what other projects they're working on. If these guys are involved, it must because they view Mason as a threat."

"How am I going to do that? A lot of that information is locked down. Isn't it?"

"You know anyone inside?"

"No."

"Then go there."

"Go there? Are you crazy?"

"Not at all. Look, I can help. I've got a couple of pals from business school who are investment bankers. Their analysts do it all the time."

"You've got to be kidding."

"I'm not. It's a lot easier than you think. Can you act?"

"What?"

"Just act. You don't have a choice. Mason's about to take a lot of heat. The public wants to hang him and if there's something there… Besides, you're the only one who knows what to look for. You know the most about Mason's research."

Hawthorn sat back down on one of the twin beds. "This is crazy." But he knew McAfee was right. He had no choice. It was the only way to help Mason. It was time to make a decision. He was faced with risking everything if this didn't work: his future, his fiancée, his parent's money put up for him to go to school, everything.

For the next two hours, they worked the logistics of what would need to happen. McAfee would call ahead to arrange a tour of Geniomics' research and development division. He would explain that "Darren Bass" was a young fund manager directly in charge of selecting biotech stocks for inclusion in a new high-growth fund. His intentions were to better acquaint himself with the R&D projects that held promise for the future of his fund investors.

Hawthorn would leave for Seattle in approximately thirty-six hours. This would give him enough time to find a flight, produce documentation for references, and confirm time away from the hospital.

In the end, both agreed it was the right thing to do. Hawthorn's father had told him long ago that in the depths of adversity, greatness is born. With this in mind, Hawthorn moved forward, determined to not give up on Mason, his research, or his father's life. The two men shook hands and left the hotel. There was a lot of work to do and time was running short.

CHAPTER TWENTY-FIVE

Mrs. Rose slept in peaceful silence as a monitor high above her head cast a whitish glow through midnight darkness in her hospital room. It'd been nearly two hours since the last nurse's visit and her frail body remained motionless beneath a thin white sheet that was pulled high around her neck and tucked neatly into the sides of the mattress. Several tubes rose from beneath the bed like fiber optic vines only to disappear again beneath the sheets.

The door cracked open allowing the pale hallway light to gradually illuminate the room. Like a dark shadow, the figure of a man slipped into the suite and quietly closed the door.

He then moved around the edge of the bed, stopping momentarily next to the monitor. His eyes swept over the sleeping woman as he reached out and traced the features of her face with a gloved hand that danced inches from her skin. He paused near her breast where he grasped a small cross attached to her necklace. He examined it, flipping it over and over in his hand, and then carefully hid it beneath a loose part of her hospital gown.

The intruder then turned his attention to the respirator. Again, his hand floated across the control panel without touching any of the buttons. His finger followed the beeping sounds of the pulse monitor.

He pulled back his sleeve and looked at his watch, an expensive, silver Bavarian. He squeezed both sides of the timepiece and the numbers began to change rapidly in the display. He looked at the respirator and turned the power off.

For the first few moments there was no reaction as the remaining oxygen pushed through the tubes and into Mrs. Rose's lungs. Fifteen seconds later, her chest fell for the last time and small dots of light began to speed across the screen.

Blip. Blip. Blip. Blip. Blip.

With death eminently approaching, Mrs. Rose's expression remained unchanged. The only indication that anything was wrong was the increasing beat of the pulse monitor. The intruder looked again to his timepiece, paying close attention to the quickly changing numbers. The vital monitor was connected electronically to the nurses' station, which meant that one of the night orderlies would be arriving soon.

Blip. Blip. Blip. Blip. Bleeeeeeeeeeeeeep.

It was over. The man reached quickly to the monitor's screen and navigated through two touch-tone menus, pressing a button labeled "set test levels."

*   *   *   *   *   *   *   *

A small red light flashed rapidly beneath the vacant nurse's desk. Soon, the pulsating lights had grown in number as the red bulb was joined by a yellow and then a blue.

As the array of bulbs flashed their concern, two evening nurses laughed and joked with each other in a small break room behind a wall of glass. A small radio played loudly in the background as one of the nurses lip-synched to the music.

James, one of the evening orderlies, emerged from the small break room taking a large bite from a slice of pizza. He walked over to a small counter where he began to pick a number of black olives into the nearby trashcan. Then he heard the buzzing. And then he saw the red light. And the yellow. Then blue. He dropped his plate on the counter and yelled back into the small room, "Gina!"

*   *   *   *   *   *   *   *

The intruder rapidly reset the machine's test levels to those matching Mrs. Rose's original settings. The first setting placed the O2 count. Next, the pulse readout was set to exactly mimic her heart rate. Then the respirator was turned back on and the visual graph on the screen showed Mrs. Rose's normal breathing pattern. As if she were suddenly alive, her chest began to rise and fall.

As the man leaned over to avoid a tube traveling from the IV stand to the woman's wrist, a stethoscope and pen slid from his front pocket and emptied onto the floor beneath the bed. Panicked, the man stooped and stretched his hand far beneath the bed frame to pick up the pen, practically pushing his face to bed frame and scrounging the floor blindly with an open palm.

Suddenly, the man jerked back with pain. He'd caught the top part of his hand on a screw's jagged metal edge, tearing a large hole through the glove and into the skin. The off-white rubber filled quickly with human blood.

*   *   *   *   *   *   *   *

Both nurses exploded from the small room carrying an assortment of equipment. James burst past the desk and into the empty hallway.

"James, wait."

He stopped. The second attendant was staring at the indicator panel on the main desk.

"390?"

"Yeah. 390. Dr. Shane's. Let's go."

"It's off."

"What?"

"Bulbs are normal. Nothing's flashing."

"I just heard the p-alarm. 390. Look at the lights."

"Yeah. 390. Nothing. Come take a look."

James jogged to the edge of the desk and looked at the panel. All of the lights had returned to normal and a small screen showed Mrs. Rose's vitals.

"I'll check it out. Just to make sure."

Within seconds James entered the dark room. Everything looked normal. Oxygen count looked good. Pulse normal. Satisfied, he exited the room allowing Mrs. Rose plenty of time to sleep.

PROPHECY

CHAPTER TWENTY-SIX

Nearly twenty years ago, in a third-world hospital at the base of Mt. Kilamanjaro, Dr. Williams lost his wife to cancer. Her one request to him was that she be able to see the savannas of South-Central Africa before she passed away. And despite the incredibly intense pain she endured to get there, her dream finally came true. On the tenth night, in a makeshift hospital bed, she took her last breaths of life.

She meant everything to him, and in the years following her death, Williams dedicated himself fully to his career and to the Center he would call his own. He always told his colleagues that without the Center, he'd be lost again. As time progressed, however, hospital protocols and technology changed. Doctors no longer cared about the patient, they now looked at dollar figures on which to base their success. The name of the game was patient turnover; move 'em in and move 'em out. The closer he came to retirement, the more he was faced with preparing for a life alone, both financially and socially. The world had passed him by and he knew it. But he wouldn't go down without a fight. He still had his Center. His focus shifted away from the treatment of patients and towards building a larger stake in the CME. Towards building a strong financial cushion. He had to look out for himself.

Despite the seemingly gigantic publicity problems now facing the hospital, Williams slept as peacefully as a newborn. He'd finally turned the corner. All angles had been covered. Even if the news report wasn't enough for the investigative committee to suspend Mason from his research in the next two days, Williams' unmarked package now en route to Mason's home would surely do the trick. Retirement was only a year away and, with Mason out of the picture, his golden years would truly be golden.

The sound of his phone woke him from a deep slumber.

"Yes?"

"Dr. Williams?" It sounded like someone from the hospital.

"Yes," he answered, clearing his throat. An alarm clock next to the phone read: 4:15 a.m.

"Uh, Dr. Williams, I think you may want to come down to the center. We have another situation here."

Williams threw off the sheets and turned on a nearby lamp. "Situation?"

"Yes. It's, well, sir, it's another of Dr. Shane's patients."

"Who knows about this?"

"Excuse me?"

"Who on staff is aware of this situation?"

"I don't know. Besides myself, one, maybe two nurses. The place is pretty empty."

"I'll be there in twenty minutes. No one is to know about this. It's a very delicate situation. I'll take care of it when I get there."

"Uh, there's one more thing, doctor."

"What?"

"We found something in the room."

"What do you mean?"

"It's a stethoscope."

"I'll be there shortly. No one's to touch that room. Am I clear?"

"Yes, sir. Should we call the police?"

"No. Not yet. Just wait for me to get there."

Williams hung up the phone and looked blankly at the floor. A small alarm clock ticked forward at a snail's pace. He finally realized what was happening. He picked up the phone and dialed Edmonds at home.

"Hello?" Edmonds answered, barely coherent.

"Randy, you promised me no one would be touched. You gave me your word."

"Allen, what time is it? Calm down."

"You calm down, Randy. What do you think you're doing? You think this helps my situation? You think the public isn't going to eat this up?"

"Allen, please. The money wasn't working. And your committee was stalling. Three days, Allen. Three days and we win. Think of it as insurance."

"At- at first I thought it was a blessing to have him losing two patients."

"It is."

"Who's responsible?"

"I think it's better you not concern yourself with that."

Williams was enraged. "This has gone way too far, Randy. Do you understand me? Way too far."

"Well let me clue you in on something, my dear friend. You're in. Whether you like it or not, you-are-in. I gave you enough ammunition today to drive a stake through the heart of this guy. And don't try to give me some sermon on morality. You're in this for one reason, Allen. Money and greed. Pure and simple. You need it worse than anyone and don't you forget it. You better get your head together, cause you-are-in pal. All the way. Call me when you clear your thoughts."

The line went dead.

*   *   *   *   *   *   *   *

The head nurse met Williams near the lobby's front doors at precisely 4:35 a.m. From there he was escorted to room 390 where Mrs. Rose lay peacefully in an eternal sleep. All of her tubes had been removed and each machine turned off except for the vital signs monitor that continued to show her heartbeat, O2 count, and breathing readouts.

Williams was shown the stethoscope lying slightly beneath the bed. He dropped to a knee and without touching the instrument, read off some numbers to the nurse who copied everything onto a blank piece of paper. Every issued piece of hospital equipment, from stethoscopes to thermometers, had a five-digit code on them that could be traced back to the practicing physician or nurse. Of course it created extra paperwork, but Williams felt everyone must be held accountable for their actions especially if something went wrong.

Williams slipped on a pair of gloves and carefully grabbed the ends of the stethoscope with the tips of his fingers. The nurse held out a small plastic bag as he slid the evidence inside. He then turned his attention to the monitor staring closely at the changing graphs.

"I've never seen anything like it, Dr. Williams. Everything on the panel at the nurses' station was normal. Everything. There's no way we missed it."

Williams was busy traveling though page after page on the touch-screen program. After four or five menus he reached the 'set test' menu where he entered his five-digit physician ID code to gain access. Someone had set the machine to run tests for ten hours.

"I didn't even know that menu existed," said the nurse. Williams' greatest fear was that some underling would accidentally hit the 'set test' button while a patient was hooked up. He'd called the manufacturer to have a security option installed as part of the purchase price.

More importantly, Beltman had designed the network architecture such that each physician would have the same five-digit code for most security measures around the hospital. Whoever was doing Edmonds' dirty work was a hospital employee or at least had a code.

"We believe it was another cardiac arrest. The only physician we could find was Dr. Briggs. He ran a couple of tests and then recommended we call you before taking any further actions."

"Her O2?" Williams asked. He was staring at the test settings.

The nurse picked the patient's file up from a meal tray and said, "Looks like seventy-nine."

Williams looked at the setting: 79. The rest of the settings matched as well.

"Would you like for me to notify the authorities now, sir?"

"No. No. I'll take care of that myself," Williams answered, exiting the room. The nurse handed him the plastic bag and the patient's file. "Can you make the arrangements here?"

The nurse nodded.

"I want your word that nothing of this situation is leaked. I anticipate some changes will be made when we find out what happened here."

"Of course, Dr. Williams."

*   *   *   *   *   *   *   *

At six fifteen, Brenner was asked to report immediately to the hospital. All Williams told her was that there was a serious situation calling for her attendance without delay.

"What's this all about, Allen?" she asked apprehensively, slipping through his door.

He took a deep breath and turned off his computer. "It's Mason."

"What? Oh, no. Not another-"

Williams put on his square reading glasses and opened the patient file on his desk. "Mrs. Angelica Rose. Age eighty-six. Grandmother of ten it says here.

Admittance was for an allergic reaction to some antibiotics. Room 390. You're more than welcome to look at it if you'd like."

Brenner slumped into a chair as Williams read the rest of her diagnosis and case history. As he expected, she appeared both shocked and disheartened.

When he finished, Williams sat the plastic bag on top of his desk. "This is what I'm sure you'll find most revealing of all." He pushed the bag towards the desk's edge as she stood to examine it. "Provisions matched ID numbers with that of Dr. Shane. This is his stethoscope."

Brenner looked over the package silently and then said, "Just because his stethoscope was found there-"

"Sarah, please. I know how much he means to you, but this time it's pretty clear. Dr. Shane is involved whether you like it or not. We also have proof that he accessed the vitals monitor and changed some of the settings. His security badge was used to gain access to several levels of the hospital ten minutes before and five minutes after."

Williams could tell Brenner had all but given up. There was no way she could argue anymore. Regardless of his methods, Edmonds had finally given Williams the evidence he'd needed all along. Whether or not Mason was guilty was no longer the issue; Brenner and her committee could no longer support Dr. Shane. Mason would have to be suspended as soon as possible for the safety of the Center.

"Have you contacted him?" she asked softly.

Williams shook his head. "No."

"What about the police?"

"No. I wanted to speak with you first." Williams stood and walked around the corner of his desk. "Sarah, if I call the police, Dr. Shane will undoubtedly go to jail. The public will feed on it like a pack of hungry sharks. His career will be ruined. The CME, too, will suffer. We both know it'd be impossible to recruit the same level of talent and funding if the Center's reputation was tainted publicly."

Williams folded his arms and glanced outside through the window. "I have no idea if he was involved in the previous two deaths, and to tell you the truth, right now that is not my concern. What is my concern, however, is that Mason is directly linked to this one."

Brenner gazed at the floor as Williams continued.

"We both agree that Mason is a brilliant researcher. His status in this industry is unquestioned. Clearly, he has a lot to offer the world. For all we know he may have what it takes to cure cancers of every kind. We also both know that this woman... Mrs. Rose... was about to die. She would have lived another two, maybe three weeks, tops. What I'm trying to tell you, Sarah, is that I'm willing to look the other way on this to save both the center and Dr. Shane's career, as long as he's suspended until things die down and we can truly gauge the extent of what's going on here."

"You asking if I think we should-"

"That's right. Bury it. I'm leaving it up to you."

Brenner shook her head and then retracted, wavering a bit on the thought. She understood the situation. "Fine," she said. "We'll suspend him. No police."

Williams nodded his head approvingly. "Good. I think it's the right thing to do. If it turns out he had nothing to do with it then we'll gladly invite him back. In the meantime, however, I think we'll spare him much heartache by not going to the authorities."

Brenner stood and quietly walked towards the door.

"Sarah," he called out. "He'll be here at 7:30."

She gave no reply and slowly closed the door.

For Williams, the final straw had been drawn. By burying the evidence, he avoided both negative publicity as well as potential lawsuits resulting from a negligent employee. Most importantly, Mason would finally be separated from his research. The ball was rolling and the landscape was all downhill.

*   *   *   *   *   *   *   *

Like a prisoner of war, Mason stood solitary before the mighty investigative committee. A panel of seven physicians sat along a polished wood table with their arms crossed and their gazed fixed on his mangled appearance.

"Please sit down, Dr. Shane," Williams said dryly.

Mason slouched into a lone chair. His face was narrowed and pale from the lack of food and sleep over the last four days.

"How are you feeling, Dr. Shane? Better, I hope."

Williams had already assigned most of his patients to other physicians in anticipation of this day.

"Can we get this over with?" A couple of panel members doubtfully shook their heads. One crossed his arms and whispered something in another man's ear.

Williams grinned. "By all means, Dr. Shane. By all means. We'll get right to the point." He flipped over the first page of a thick report and each member followed in synch. "Early this morning, at approximately 1:22 a.m., Mrs. Rose in 390 passed away."

"She died, did she?" Mason asked. He chuckled as if he were not surprised.

"Yes, Dr. Shane. Four hours ago. Cardiac arrest."

"Unbelievable."

"Very believable, unfortunately, Dr. Shane. As of this time, by the recommendation of the investigative committee here before you, you are suspended from all hospital duties. You will continue to receive benefits until you have been reaffirmed. One month from now your reinstatement will be considered."

"Do you really think I've done something wrong?"

"Your patients are dying, doctor. I'd say something's wrong."

"Really? Then let me ask you this- and any of you can answer if you like. Is death a means to freedom?"

No one answered, each face casting an empty gaze upon him.

"Imagine you're Mrs. Rose, hooked up to all those machines. You can't eat, you can't communicate to your family... you can't even breath the air around you. Each day is spent in a spiraling slumber, slowly closing down the human clock within."

"Mason-" Brenner interrupted. Williams put his hand on her arm allowing Mason to continue. Dig your hole, Mason.

"Then you have us: life saving heroes desperately trying to salvage her life. For what? Are we rescuing her or prolonging her suffering? When that woman passed away, she achieved freedom. Freedom from tubes poking holes throughout her body. Freedom from medication forced upon her. And freedom from a daily audience of strangers monitoring her decay. That woman was set free."

"A fascinating perspective, Dr. Shane. Is there anything else you'd like to share with us?"

"I have nothing left to say."

"I'm sorry to hear that, Dr. Shane. Does anyone have anything to add?" Everyone shook their heads. "Then this meeting is over."

CHAPTER TWENTY-SEVEN

Hawthorn rummaged quietly through his locker, careful not to disturb Dr. Xiao who sat in a recliner with his back to the rest of the physician's lounge. Other than midnight, high noon was Xiao's favorite time of day, everyone out eating lunch and he with the physicians' lounge all to himself. Hawthorn figured it was the only time when Xiao could rise from the depths of the basement floor and avoid the usual glares from the daily staff. It was a time when he could frame himself in the path of a large window, letting the afternoon sun warm his pale skin while he jogged merrily through the gory illustrations of the latest journal on pathology.

Xiao arrived at the end of a long paragraph and then marked his place in the passage. He shut the book's cover and cocked his head back into the thick cushions of the recliner, slowly closing his thin eyes as if to concentrate on the full warmth of the sun.

The calmness on Xiao's face was more than Hawthorn could handle. "Strange world when everything around you breathes, huh?"

Xiao dropped the magazine to his lap and spun his chair sideways to face Hawthorn. "Would you like me to see your patients, Hawthorn? After all, they'll be mine soon."

Hawthorn threw his foot up on the edge of a small stool, retying his shoe. "Prepare to wait a long time. We're not giving up on anybody up here."

"Oh? What about Mrs. Rose, Hawthorn? Somebody gave up on her."

"What are you talking about?" he asked, fumbling with the shoestrings.

"Let's just say she's no longer with us."

"I'm not in the mood for jokes."

"Me neither, Hawthorn. It amuses me to watch you wage war against the inevitable. Heart and soul poured into each patient, and what? The end result always the same."

"My job is to ease the patient's suffering, not give them immortality."

"Is that what your friend Dr. Shane did? He tried to ease that patient's suffering and now he's out of a job."

Hawthorn pulled his laces tight. "What?"

"He was suspended early this morning, John. I thought you'd know that. It's doctors like the two of you keep me in business." Hawthorn stopped what he was doing and stared Xiao down as if the next move would be physical. "Go ahead, Hawthorn. Join him."

Hawthorn thought better of it and continued angrily gathering his things. "Who suspended him?"

"Williams. And a committee of some sort."

"Where is he? Have you seen Mason?"

Xiao rolled the magazine up into his hand and walked towards the door. "Mason? Oh, I'm sure he'll turn up somewhere. They always do."

*　　*　　*　　*　　*　　*　　*　　*

Hawthorn rapped loudly on Brenner's door. He couldn't believe she'd allow this to happen. She'd always been there for Mason. For her to do this must have meant that the committee found something even she couldn't turn away.

"Come in, John," she said, leading him into her office. "I can imagine why you're here."

"I'm sure you can."

"I appreciate what you're trying to do, but given the recent events concerning his patients, we really had no other alternative. It's in the best interest of the center."

"This is crazy. You know as well as I do that there is no other professional in the hospital who performs at the same level as Mason. This place has consistently beaten him down simply because he wants to pursue research. He has always treated each patient with the utmost care. Always."

"I couldn't agree with you more. I also know you're his friend and you're trying to help. But, really. There was nothing else for us to do."

"There's got to be a mistake here. How can you suspend him without incriminating evidence? There's no way Mason would hurt anyone."

"Look, John. We share many of the same concerns but, as one of the hospital's directors, I have certain responsibilities. One of them is to protect the center's good name. You can understand that."

"So you suspend him without evidence?"

Brenner looked him square in the eye and said, "It's in the best interest of the hospital. That's all I can say."

Hawthorn walked to the edge of her desk, picking up a small copper paperweight shaped like a deer. He ran his fingers down the back its head, feeling each and every horn poke beneath his fingers.

"He's in trouble," Hawthorn said gravely. He sat the tiny statuette back in its place. "He doesn't eat, he doesn't sleep, I can't get a hold of him at his house-"

"Where does he go?" she asked.

"The library? Out of town? To tell you the truth, I really don't know."

"Should we call someone for him?"

"No," said Hawthorn. "That won't do any good. He won't listen to me, let alone a stranger."

"Please. The committee just needs time to let things die down a bit. We both know that public and industry perception is a big part of the game here."

"Perception? Who cares about that. Dr. Brenner, we're talking about irreversible damage to his career."

"Hawthorn, I understand."

"I just want to know why he was suspended."

"Because three of his patients have died and the hospital is being cornered in the press. It's a ball game no one wants to play, John. Including me. But it is my job. It is my duty."

Hawthorn looked her over, trying to gauge if she were telling the truth. It was impossible to tell. He had to play it safe and not say a word.

"If there was something we could do," she continued, "I would tell you. But really, John, there's nothing. A month will come and go before you know it."

"So that's it."

"What's done is done. Mason's name will be cleared tomorrow but he will be suspended until we have time to finalize these investigations."

Hawthorn lifted his clipboard from a small table located between the two chairs. "I guess you feel okay with everything."

She gave Hawthorn a scornful look. "You know I had to do it. I don't have a choice. I have to feel okay about it."

"Fine."

"I'm truly sorry, John. I hope you understand."

Hawthorn shut the door quietly behind and traveled to the third floor to finish his rounds. He figured he would go home after work, make a few phone calls, and then spend the rest of the afternoon with Jordan. First, however, he had to call McAfee to make sure everything was ready for the trip to Seattle. And then he needed to ask Cindy to cover for him on the Slvy-M measurements while he was gone. Hawthorn wanted to explain to her all that was happening. He needed a contact at the hospital. Someone he could rely on. Most importantly, he had to find Mason to make sure he was all right. No telling what was going on with him.

*   *   *   *   *   *   *   *

Mason sat cross-legged on a large, hand-woven rug in the middle of his living room floor. All of the furniture had been pushed to the far edges of the room leaving plenty of space for Mason and his materials.

The entire floor around him was covered in books ranging from Indian philosophy and religion to dream interpretation and studies on the human psyche. Several piles of cans, bottles, and food wrappings were also strewn about the room.

Directly before him was a blank pad of paper and a black ink pen. He closed his eyes and relaxed in deep meditation. Slowly, his hand elevated from his side and took hold of the pen. He straightened his arm and carefully drew what at first looked like a backwards 'S'. The shape soon changed as other lines crossed its curves at various points, some curving and some remaining straight.

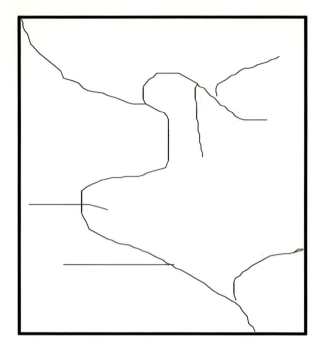

With his eyes closed, Mason marked each intersecting line with a two-letter abbreviation. Occasionally he would label one of the lines with a single letter or a number.

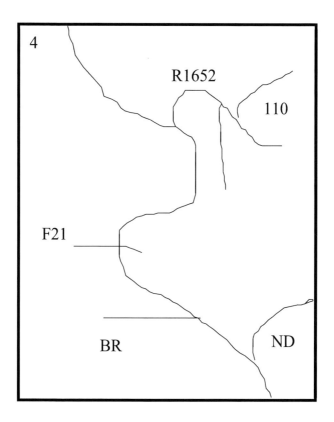

When he finished, Mason slowly opened his eyes and reached deep into his shirt pocket, withdrawing the small folded note found earlier in the Old County library.

Carefully, Mason unfolded the note and placed it directly on top of the figure just drawn, making sure the edges of the two pieces were placed neatly together. Wiping the sweat from his brow, Mason could see that the map he had drawn from memory matched the original line for line.

CHAPTER TWENTY-EIGHT

Edmonds opened the day with a special news conference downtown proudly stating that Geniomics had passed its final test. Close to one hundred news people and journalists from leading stations packed the small suite, each armed with lists of probing questions. Edmonds had instructed the Geniomics staff members to do everything short of physically massaging members of the press in order to initiate a positive outlook for his company. There were fabulous refreshments, large Geniomics banners, and handshakes from just about anyone associated with the firm.

"Excuse me, ladies and gentlemen," said a young spokeswoman for the company. Most of the reporters were still hovering around the magnificent tray of food in the back. "Excuse me. Thank you."

One by one, the row of cameras in the back of the room powered up their bright lights. The young woman spoke from a raised stage with a small podium mounted at its front. Attached to the podium were eight or nine microphones labeled with four letter station codes. All the big ones were there. Draped behind her was a huge blue and white banner that cradled the Geniomics logo and read: Caring for our Future.

"Ladies and Gentlemen, I present to you Geniomics' Founder, CEO and Chairman of the Board, Randy Edmonds." The reporters shuffled their materials one last time as Edmonds took the stand.

"Good morning, and thank you all for coming. As you know, one of our largest competitors in the market, Triton Corporation, announced yesterday that they believe their R2-X clone tests are nearing completion. Apparently the experts down on Wall Street are interpreting it as bad news for Geniomics. I guess they know more about drug discovery than us."

There were a few chuckles from the crowd.

"The reason I called this conference today is to let those experts know that, as of last night, we have passed our fourth and final test for the approval of R2-X and we eagerly anticipate immediate, worldwide availability. Seven days after FDA approval our product will on your neighborhood shelves. I am proud to announce that the cure for the common cold will be available to everyone in the world in just over one week."

Edmonds put on his best fake smile and the crowd erupted into questioning.

"Are you concerned that, with Triton apparently sharing the market, your profits will be much less than expected?" a woman asked from the back row.

Edmonds smiled. "Fair question. The answer is 'no'. Our distribution system is light years ahead of theirs and stands ready to bring product to market a mere week following approval."

"What about the scale of your investment?" asked another woman in the back. "Are you betting too much on this drug?"

"Every person in the world suffers from a cold on the average of two times per year – productivity lost and human suffering can barely be measured. We are not betting too much. All of our risks are calculated and conservative. We anticipate our highest profits ever for each of the next five quarters, even if Triton is in the market."

Edmonds went on to praise his R&D division as the most efficient in history while reinforcing that Geniomics anticipated no problems gaining market approval from the FDA. Only a few select people, including Dr. Williams, knew the truth.

According to an inside source at Triton, their R&D had come up with a formula using abundant synthetic and natural materials. By the time Geniomics realized Triton's approach the investments had been made. For Geniomics, no enzyme equaled no FDA approval. Edmonds would be on the cover of TIME for all the wrong reasons.

After the conference, Edmonds spent lunch at Salty's, a seafood restaurant eight minutes from downtown that offered a spectacular view of the Seattle skyline. Many CEO's in the high-tech community frequented the establishment to talk business or relax with people sharing similar headaches.

Edmonds swirled his drink around once or twice and finished it off. A waitress brought a cup of coffee and placed it in front of Crooks.

"How do you feel about this morning?" Edmonds asked.

"Nervous."

"I think things went well, though. Don't you?"

"We'll have that answer in a few minutes." The two men were supposed to hear from Camden in marketing any minute.

Edmonds smiled and waved to a Microsoft executive at a distant table. "You think Triton's bluffing?"

Crooks shrugged his shoulders. "Hard to say. I doubt it. They're killing themselves if they announce with no product. We don't have a choice but to believe them."

Edmonds cell phone rang loudly from beneath the confines of his jacket. "Yep."

"Hello, Randy. This is Camden."

Crooks raised his eyebrows and waited eagerly from across the table.

"Yeah, go ahead."

"Up six and three eights," Camden said dolefully. "No change from Triton. They're committed to the 24th."

Crooks watched the stress in Edmonds face disappear into a look of surprise. "My God, Camden, lighten up. You make it sound like your mom just died. That uptick alone just made you one point two mill." Edmonds put his hand over the receiver and quietly mouthed, "Up six."

"We also signed that Japanese account and the Chinese are right behind them."

"You're kidding. The Chinese are finally coming on board? Well, congratulations to you and the rest of the marketing staff. Take them to dinner."

Edmonds hung up the phone and placed it back inside his jacket. "See? I told you. No harm done. Everyone's happy."

Crooks shook his head. "There's a long way to go."

Edmonds leaned forward, quieting his voice. "I'm going to order Phase II."

"What?! No, Randy. I don't know if that's a good idea."

"Of course it is. Think of what it'll do for our production schedule. That gives us six additional days. Start production now and we'll have product on the shelves one day after approval. The market will shit their pants."

"Randy, you're talking about putting a drug on the market that could make a lot of people sick. Need I remind you-" Crooks looked nervously around the room. "We've yet to pass L-4. For six lousy days? Is it really worth it?"

"Please," snapped Edmonds. "We both know those tests will be passed." He leaned back in his chair, basking in gallant delight. "We're gonna leapfrog those bastards."

Crooks was shaking his head. "We don't know-"

"We're close enough on those tests as it is," Edmonds exclaimed. "Think of the people- Christ, I'm talking six days."

"But the drug isn't ready. And R3-X is unproven in the animal models. We're not ready."

"What are our latest test numbers for L-4?"
Edmonds asked, falling back into his know-it-all mode.
"Go ahead. Tell me."

"Randy, that's not the point."

"You know what they are. Two percent as of today.
Let's run through the numbers, Wally. You're the
Goddamn numbers guy. Ten thousand people get a cold
and take R2-X. Two hundred develop varying degrees of
complications and nine thousand eight hundred get cured.
Within the first week, we get the tests down to less than one
tenth and now only ten in ten thousand get sick. How can
we look the other way?"

"You want to break the law for six extra days? No
way. I say it's not worth it. People may die."

"Of course it's worth it. I'm talking finished
product on the shelves a week earlier than originally
planned. Wall Street will love it. And we have three years
to shore up R3-X."

"The board will never-"

"The board? I tell those suit-heads what I want to
tell them. They believe what I want them to believe and
they see what I allow them to see. Why? Because they're
bags of organs and I have a brain and vision. Oxygen
thieves. Jesus, they have their own companies and
headaches. Besides, I couldn't tell you the last time I talked
to any of them. Last meeting- what, six months ago?"

Edmonds slurped though the ice in his drink as he
kept one eye on Crooks. He could tell Crooks was busy
doing the numbers in his head. Six extra days meant a ton
of money to the company. The cycle time for the
production of R2-X was about four days. Starting now
would put them on track for a worldwide launch one day
after approval. Phase II would ramp up production and
kick Triton's ass. Besides, the Macaba plant was ready to
rock and roll. The risk was a no brainer.

CHAPTER TWENTY-NINE

Jordan glanced at the clock and then slumped despairingly back into the cushions of Hawthorn's couch. At two she'd watched a talk show on men who were women who wished they were men. At two thirty another show concerning celebrities who despised fortune and fame. The last show finally did her in. Lodged deep between two blue pillows and an afghan blanket, Jordan finally drifted to sleep.

*　　*　　*　　*　　*　　*　　*　　*

Hawthorn entered his apartment and found the television blaring with an orchestra of cereal components spread out across the coffee table. He turned off the television and sat his things quietly on the chair. From across the small living room he could see the red light on his answering machine flashing rapidly.

Hawthorn moved lightly past Jordan and turned down the volume. He moved to the kitchen and gently tapped the answer machine.

"Two thirty-two," it declared.

"John, this is Mac. I've got to ask you something about a business idea I have in mind. Call me. Hi Jordan."

"Nice cover," he thought.

"Three forty-five."

The next message was from Hawthorn's mother, telling him that his father had fallen and hurt his hip. The doctor had come out and it was just a bruise. Hawthorn wondered what he'd tell them.

"Four fifteen."

"Hawthorn," Mason's voice bellowed. "Five o'clock. Old Calvary. And the truth shall set you free."

Hawthorn picked up the phone and dialed Mason's home. As usual, it rang until the answering machine picked up.

"You're late," Jordan said from the living room couch.

"I know. I'm sorry." Hawthorn quickly reset the machine.

"What time is it?

"Four thirty."

"Four thirty? And you're just getting in? I've been waiting here for three hours?"

"Please, Jordan, not now. I've had a very rough day." Hawthorn crossed the kitchen with a jar of mayonnaise in his hand.

"I was hoping we could spend some time together. One of these days, huh, John?"

"I know. I'm sorry. I really am. I'm just very pinched for time right now."

"Time? Who do you think you're talking to here? I'm not some-"

"Jordan? Let's not do this, okay?" He was standing at the edge of the kitchen with his arms out to his sides. "I'm so busy right now, I can barely frickin breathe."

"You know what?"

"What?"

"You are a fool. A fool, John. I'm here to be with you and you're off doing- I- I don't even know what. I haven't had one single moment to talk to you and you're out screwing around. You are really threatening this entire thing. You think I want to live like this? You think I want my life to be like this? I love you but wake up. Because I have had enough."

Hawthorn caught himself before he said anything stupid. He walked over to the edge of the couch and affectionately ran his fingers through her hair as she quickly turned away. "I'm sorry," he said apologetically. "Another of Mason's patients passed away last night."

Jordan spun beneath his arm. "Another? Who?"

"An elderly woman named Mrs. Rose."

"How?"

"No one knows."

"And Mason?"

"Suspended. And no one can find him. We've called his house and left messages. He wants me to meet him somewhere in a few minutes." There was no way he was going to tell her where.

"I'm sorry to hear that."

"Williams' is so pissed right now, he can hardly see straight."

Jordan shifted back into the couch, allowing Hawthorn to lie beside her. He stared blankly into the ceiling, his mind racing over Mrs. Rose's hospital stay and each of the visits he and Mason had performed. He recollected every document written, each test carried out and each conversation. There were no easy answers.

"Is this what it's going to be like to be married to a doctor?" Jordan asked. "I mean, is this what I have to look forward to in five years?"

"No. Everything will calm down soon." One way or another, he thought. He kissed her lightly and walked over to the recliner. He reached into his bag and withdrew a short stem yellow rose. "I'm truly sorry, Jordan."

"John," she said, half angry and half forgiving. "Why do you always wait until the last minute to do the right thing?" She took the flower and lifted it to take in the sweet aroma of the freshly cut flower.

"I know you want to talk to me about something important. Believe me, I know this is ridiculous, but there's some very serious things going on at the center and… I want to hear what you have to say. I mean I really want to hear what you have to say. It means everything to me. You mean everything to me. When I get back. Okay?"

She smiled and said, "Okay."

*   *   *   *   *   *   *   *

As Hawthorn pulled into the small cemetery parking lot, he noticed Mason's car parked against the old, gated entrance. Chills ran down his arms as his own vehicle rolled slowly to a stop. This particular graveyard was located ten miles outside of Portland and was accessible only through a primitive dirt road. To his surprise, there were two other vehicles in the lot. Site-seers, probably. Perhaps families tracing back their roots.

Hawthorn looked to the sky. The late afternoon sun was perhaps an hour from disappearing beneath the horizon. He then walked across the dirt lot and around the side of Mason's car to the gated entrance. A thick rusted chain weaved its way between rusted iron bars and then connected at both ends to an old padlock.

Spanning the top of the gate was a rusted wrought iron arch, reading: Calvary Cemetery. Hawthorn had read about this place. Its first deposit was made in the late 1800's during the northwest gold rush. As the mineral pools began to die, so did the surrounding community. Rumor had it some of the cemetery's residents were wealthy gold miners buried with half their fortune. Many of the graves had been dug up several times by bandits following mythical tales. Since then, the state of Oregon deemed the site a historic monument meaning the cemetery's days of entertaining permanent visitors were long gone.

Twenty yards beyond the front gate's vertical bars, Hawthorn could see the tops of the first row of headstones. The pathway had long been covered with grass and vines that crept their way across the tombstones and up into the trees. Beneath their branches and to the back of the cemetery, the earth was dark as night.

"Mason!" Hawthorn yelled. His voice echoed through the forested grounds. He yelled again but there was no answer.

Hawthorn placed his hand on one of the thick iron bars. It felt sturdy. The perimeter appeared outlined by a waist high, weathered iron fence. Hawthorn leaned back to see if there was a large enough opening for him to fit.

Suddenly, the chain rattled through the bars making a loud clanking sound. Hawthorn stumbled back, pulling the gate along with him until the chain had slipped entirely through the bars and he had fallen to the ground.

Hawthorn wiped the rust from his shirt and looked nervously through the cemetery's open doors. Somehow, with the gate now open, he felt more vulnerable. His senses seemed to instantly heighten as if he could suddenly feel the slightest turn of the wind, the smallest movements in the trees.

He glanced to his car and then moved cautiously into a world unchanged for a half century. Hawthorn had never been one to scare easily. On the contrary, it was he who frightened the other kids throughout his childhood. As the gate banged closed behind him, however, Hawthorn felt instantly afraid, although from what he couldn't say. He paused at the first row of headstones. Behind them the trees began and the sunlight ended.

"Mason?"

Beneath the branches, Hawthorn could see several other headstones pushing their way through the ground. Some were the classic tombstones, square at the bottom and round at the top, and some were made of marble standing nearly six feet high. Hawthorn jumped as a blue jay flew from one tree to the next. If he was planning on finding Mason, he had to do it now.

Once beneath the trees, the temperature changed dramatically. The sun was almost entirely blocked by large fir and pine trees whose branches extended overhead, crossing each other at every possible point. Beneath their protection, the cemetery air was cool and still and offered no particular scent.

"Mason!" Hawthorn called out again.

He stepped over a series of rotted branches and several knee-high ferns scattered around the base of a tall fir. An army of thick green vines clung to its base like snakes climbing a tree. Judging from the sheer size of the tombs, Hawthorn figured he must be near the graveyard's center. He paused to wipe the sweat from his brow and suddenly his heart began to race.

Thirty yards away, Hawthorn could see a man standing at the foot of an old grave. He stepped quickly behind a nearby tree and peeked his head around the trunk's edge, peering through the gaps in the branches. It looked like Mason. Same build, same hair. Same overcoat.

When he'd finally regained control of his fear, Hawthorn quietly found his way to the main path, approaching the man from behind. "Mason?"

There was no response.

"Mason."

"Not Mason. Definitely not Mason," said Xiao. His appearance sent Hawthorn stumbling backwards.

"What are you doing here?"

"Research, John. The question is, my friend, what are you doing here?"

"I'm-"

"Looking for Mason?"

Hawthorn didn't know what to think. "Is he here?"

"Now, why would Mason be here in this distant little cemetery? It's such a small world. Isn't it?"

"Christ, Xiao. What the hell are you doing here?"

"Why, Hawthorn," said Xiao. "I love the old west. And there's nothing like a good old graveyard to brighten one's day."

"Come on, Xiao. Mason's in trouble. I need to find him. Have you seen him or not?"

"He's no concern of mine. But this may be the only place he can visit his patients now."

"Screw you."

"My. My. My," Xiao commented as he walked slowly away. "How that little tongue of yours can get away from you."

"Why can't you help for once, Xiao?"

"I help those who help themselves, Hawthorn. But in my business, it's always too late." He turned his back to Hawthorn and walked towards the exit.

"You're the most screwed up doctor I know."

Xiao stopped and spun around. "Me screwed up? You should see how low my malpractice premiums are, Hawthorn. I may be the only sane one you know." Within seconds Xiao had disappeared among the gravestones and distant trees.

Xiao's appearance fueled Hawthorn's angst. He had to be involved. What were the chances of him finding Xiao here? Then again, Xiao couldn't stand anyone long enough to be involved. Any other person would have instantly been a suspect, but Xiao?

Then again, Xiao had motive. He was Mason's nemesis, competing for the same honors in almost everything they did. The only problem was that Xiao did this sort of thing all the time. This was nothing out of character for him. He really did visit graveyards and everyone knew it.

For the next three or four minutes, Hawthorn ventured deeper into the cemetery. The sunlight above was fading and although it was only five-thirty or six o'clock, its incandescence made it seem like seven or eight.

At the end of the darkened path appeared to be a small clearing. Hawthorn reached the edge of the trees and realized he was located in the heart of the cemetery. The graveyard's center point was relatively flat with small ferns and plants springing through the ankle-high grass. Hawthorn glanced to the dim violet sky calculating how long it'd be until darkness set completely in. He had no clue where Mason could be. He could only fear the worst.

In the middle of the small clearing, a single headstone broke the ground and was surrounded by a chest-high, iron fence. Hawthorn suddenly recognized the site as the one in Mason's photograph. The iron fence profiled a plot some five hundred square feet and was joined together by a steady gate at the top of which sat a complex design displaying the word: BOONE.

Hawthorn approached the fence and ran his fingers past the design. He couldn't believe what he was doing. He'd covered a lot of ground. Mason should've at least been able to hear him call. He glanced across the gravesite to the line of trees that surrounded the clearing in a near perfect square. Between the trunks and their limbs were pockets of darkness where the cemetery extended for hundreds of yards in every direction. Anyone could be watching.

"An appropriate setting. Don't you think, Hawthorn?"

In a flash, Mason was standing directly behind him. Dressed in black pants and a black shirt, Hawthorn at first mistook him for a priest. In his right hand he held a large blue book.

"Mason," Hawthorn wavered. "Whe- Where did you come from?"

Mason ignored him and held out his hand in gentlemanly fashion. "Shall we?" he asked, indicating his intention to enter the Boone gravesite.

Hawthorn stepped aside and said, "Mason, what are we doing here? This is crazy. I need you to listen to me."

The hinges of the gate creaked loudly as Mason pried it open to allow Hawthorn safe passage. "This," he said, "is where the answers lie."

"We're in a graveyard for God's sake."

"Beautiful day, isn't it?"

Hawthorn looked at the headstone and said, "Can we please talk about this at the cars? Huh?"

"Come on," Mason said lightly. "I'd like to introduce you to someone."

Hawthorn looked around the open clearing towards the dark circle of trees. There was no one around. No one to hear him call or scream. He considered running but from his vantage point it was difficult to tell where the trail was. Several other trails met at this central location as well. For the first time, Hawthorn was beginning not to trust his good friend.

"I really don't want to do this, Mason," Hawthorn pleaded.

"Nonsense," he answered, still holding open the gate. "It takes him a while before he notices I'm here. Come on."

Hawthorn looked again at the headstone. "Mason, you need help. Please. This whole thing is not your fault. I mean, where in the hell have you been?"

Mason chuckled loudly. "Hawthorn, I too was afraid the first time I did this, but you are the only one I can trust. And I need to show this to *you*."

"Why me?"

"Because you, my friend, are a believer."

Hawthorn glanced at the trees again and then stepped just inside the gate.

Mason inhaled deeply, savoring the air as he moved quickly to the front of the headstone and promptly took a seat. "Beautiful. Beautiful day."

Hawthorn waited impatiently with one hand on the gate. He couldn't wait to get this over with.

"There was a famous general," said Mason. "Who swore he had been a soldier in each of history's greatest wars. Each time he would always be on the victorious side, each time with a slightly higher rank."

Hawthorn could barely look at Mason, his own eyes drawn constantly to the perimeter of trees.

"Each time he was born with his memory intact; always learning from his previous battles. He said it was his destiny to win. Do you believe that?"

"No," said Hawthorn. "Don't take this the wrong way, Mason, but I find it hard to believe in reincarnation of any sort."

"A cemetery is a wonderful place to reexamine your beliefs. Don't you think so, John?" Mason jumped from the tombstone and stamped his foot hard to the ground. "What do you think, Hawthorn? Can you imagine yourself down there?"

"We're all going to die someday."

"Are we?" He circled around to the back of the headstone as Hawthorn's eyes scanned over the name carved in granite: Shepard Boone. "Yes. Isn't it amazing how each of us has visited places we've never been to before, yet known with absolute certainty that we'd already been there?"

"Deja vu."

"We dismiss the feeling as if it were a trick of the mind. We do it so calmly. So casually, it's almost as if we expect it to happen."

"Mason-"

"Have you ever been to the Old County Library? It's where I've always gone to study. Even as a young man, I've always felt drawn to it. In some of the hallways where the older books are stacked, you can almost feel the ghosts walking past you. After all, a library's sort of a graveyard, isn't it?"

Hawthorn waited nervously next to the iron gate. He looked again to the sky that now glowed a deep shade of purple and blue. Wouldn't be long till he'd have to put this meeting to a close.

"I was looking through a collection of philosophical texts," Mason continued, "and that feeling suddenly came over me. I had stood beside those books in that very same spot before. Something was waiting there for me. You have to understand, John, I'd never seen any of those books before, but my hand just reached out and... viola."

Mason placed the large blue book on top of the headstone. "I sat down at a table and turned directly to a particular passage. Very interesting."

"Is that-"

"Yes. That's from where the picture came. Most interesting, however, was that lodged between these pages was a note. A message, I believe, left for me."

"From?"

Mason held up his hand. He unfolded the note and read aloud. "To whomever finds this note. I make no excuses for what I've done. Fate has not been kind to me. I was led to the path I have taken. Funny how little choice we have over the direction of our lives. I have seen many pass before me and have spoken in many voices. And always I have tried to heal the wound within me. I write these words, hoping, perhaps futily, that I will see them again when I return. When I am healed. Bearcloud is near."

Hawthorn's eyes narrowed. "Bearcloud is the spirit?"

"Yes, the dark spirit," said Mason. He pointed to the grave. "Allow me to introduce to you to Shepard Boone. This man was accused of killing two innocent people. One of the bodies was recovered, but the other never found."

Hawthorn glanced again at the headstone's face. The date of death read: January 29, 1964. There was something familiar about the date.

"You see, John, Shepard Boone left this note for me to find," Mason claimed.

Hawthorn crossed his arms. "Mason, I just feel like you're reaching for an answer."

"People were dying around him, John, and now they are dying around me."

"Mason, please, I really-"

"They questioned him, too. They questioned him and he could never remember a thing."

Hawthorn nervously checked his watch. He thought about Mason's blackouts. There was no way. Hawthorn simply would not accept it. "Look, I've really got to go."

"Wait, Hawthorn," Mason replied. "Shepard Boone died on the very day I was born: January 29, 1964. He was the last one buried here."

Hawthorn sighed. "Mason, this isn't going to help you solve your problems at the center."

"This note," Mason continued, "and these visions are proof that reincarnation is reality. Look at it," he said, slapping the back of his hand to the paper. He straightened it with his two hands and repeated the key phrase. "Have spoken in many voices. Can't you see?"

Hawthorn swallowed heavily. He didn't know what to think. At this point he just wanted to leave.

"Bearcloud lived through Boone and now he lives through me. The proof," Mason laughed, "is right in front of your eyes."

Hawthorn remained quiet. There was nothing he could do to help Mason out here.

Mason ran his fingers over the top of the gravestone and then turned his attention to the open book, his eyes skipping over some words as if he were looking for another quote. "Hawthorn, I need you to come with me."

"Where?"

"Vernonia."

"Where's that?"

"Northwest. One hour"

"I don't have time to go up there."

"Please, I'm close to understanding. I get glimpses. I've done everything to understand them. I know where to go now. This note will show me the way. You're the only one I can trust."

"Mason, I can't. I would if I had the time but I've got the hospital, and then there's Jordan- You know I would if I could. But Mason, you're just not listening to me. I mean you hear me, but you don't listen."

Hawthorn's pager buzzed loudly from the case holder attached to his belt. He withdrew the device and stared wearily into the display. It was the emergency room again. He was needed immediately. "I've got to go, Mason. Its ER."

"Emergency," repeated Mason. "An unforeseen combination of circumstances or the resulting state that calls for immediate action."

"Look, I have to go now."

"Which is the emergency John? Do you really know?"

Hawthorn had already backed out through the gate and was letting it shut slowly with his hand. "I can't go with you right now, Mason. I'm sorry. I'll talk to you as soon as I can. Please be home tonight. I'll call you right when I get home."

It was a difficult decision for Hawthorn to make. If he missed that call, his career was over. He was already on thin ice with Williams who wouldn't hesitate to remove him from his duties. On the other hand, here was his best friend, in some distant world seriously believing he may have lived previous lives. Either way someone was close to dying. Hawthorn just wasn't sure who.

CHAPTER THIRTY

For centuries, the jungles of South America served as a breeding ground for some of the most deadly creatures known to mankind. There were snakes that could squeeze a person so hard their eyeballs were forced out of their head. Scorpions that with one sting could send a grown man spiraling towards an eternal slumber. There were even schools of fish that could devour entire livestock in one eating. For centuries, these jungles offered a safe haven for world's most dreaded killers. To many, this environment meant fear and uncertainty. For Geniomics, it represented the opportunity of a lifetime.

Two of Geniomics' dock loaders waited patiently at the edge of the receiving bay, swatting constantly at the giant insects that swarmed the powerful outdoor lights. Both were dressed in yellow Gore-Tex body suits complete with an attached helmet that hung loosely behind their backs. Each was an American ex-patriot on temporary assignment in South America. It was their sole responsibility to set up the first three months of operations so that the Brazilian workers would have time to adjust to the new technology and transfer system of the R2-X facility.

The first man glanced at his watch. It was two fifteen in the morning, Macaba time, and the workers had been waiting patiently for the first shipment of the Conrava Goliath species. Behind them was a massive steel door marking the receiving bay for the entire R2-X factory.

The facility's technical complexity was fascinating. When a truck was ready to deposit its contents, the large steel door would open and the dock would slide backwards so that the truck could back up beneath the factory's roof.

To keep the frogs moist, each truck was equipped with complex, high-tech misting and temperature control systems. Once the massive trucks had backed partially beneath the building, larger misters would shoot water from the ceilings onto the small amphibians as they slid down a wide plastic chute to a holding area beneath the ground.

The purpose of the misters was to help maintain the frog's skin temperature. If their environment changed by more than five or six degrees it would mean changes in their skin temperature, and as far as Geniomics research knew, that meant certain death and money lost.

"Damn these bugs," said one of the men, swatting the air in front of his face. "Texas don't have shit on these things."

"That ain't no lie," the other man agreed. He kicked his legs back and forth as they dangled over the edge of the dock. "They're like dogs with wings."

The first man reached beneath the sleeve of his jumpsuit and pulled out a half-full pack of cigarettes. "You go into town today?"

"Hell no, Ray. Thirty minutes on this crap road? I'd rather just break my spine here and save the trip. You know who built the road, don't you?"

The other man shrugged his shoulders.

"Nationals. So our company wouldn't take the blame for clearing forest."

"That's smart."

"Yeah but it still means crap for a road."

"Didn't think we'd be receiving shipment so soon."

"Me neither," said the first man. "White coats must've passed them tests."

In the distance, the men could hear what sounded like deep, rumbling thunder. They looked up at the sky but found a cloudless night with a sparkling array of stars.

As the noise grew louder, both men bounced to their feet and threw their cigarettes to the ground. The first worker grabbed his clipboard, which held a printout detailing the delivery schedule. Three quarters of a mile down the road, at the first major turn, a white glow could be seen slowly growing in intensity. "First shipment ain't for another two hours. What the hell is that?"

The other man shrugged his shoulders.

A side door opened and out walked Ted Malley, Geniomics' South American Director of Operations. Each worker straightened their posture as Malley walked beside them. He carried with him three pairs of noise reduction headphones.

"Enjoying the show?" he asked, speaking loudly to overtake the distant, booming noise.

"What is it?" one of the men inquired.

Malley nodded towards the glow and said, "Watch. You're about to witness technological might."

The glow at the end of the road seemed to peak in intensity when suddenly powerful lights blinded the men. Malley handed each man a pair of headphones, which they immediately placed over their ears.

In a matter of minutes, the powerful lights had grown in number to three, then four, and now five. Every ten seconds or so another brilliant light would appear causing each person to cover their eyes as if they were blocking out the direct rays of the setting sun.

The plant's powerful outdoor lights flashed several times behind them, and like a set of dominoes, the singular lights in the distance shut down one by one. It was then that the two loaders could see the perimeter lights outlining the huge fleet of Selva trucks. The vehicles were massive, one tire measuring ten feet tall. From the ground to the top part of the cab was over twenty-five feet. Geniomics had adapted them for the temperature sensitive transport of the frogs across jungle terrain. Each cost in excess of five million dollars and could never be transported to any other part of the world.

*   *   *   *   *   *   *   *

Malley saw the first man look again to his charts. His numbers would tell him there were only supposed to be three cargo loads. The most they were ever supposed to entertain was five in one twenty-four hour shift. That was what the Conservation Consortium had made into international law.

The worker looked up from his charts and made a visual count of the trucks. He glanced to Malley who returned the look with a stale nod.

Like a family of elephants, the string of trucks made a giant circle to back into the individual docking bays. The massive receiving door broke from its base and rose slowly behind them, exposing the large interior slots. Malley nodded for his men to place the hoods over their heads. Once the massive door had locked into its open position, hundreds of misters began to spray water over the entire area.

Yellow and red lights flashed all around as several workers dressed in waterproof jumpsuits entered the bays from multiple side doors. Some of them rolled the massive chutes into position as others helped guide the trucks into their slots. Though his American team appeared to be executing in near perfect fashion, Malley was anything but satisfied.

Earlier that day, he'd been involved in a conference call to a European warehouse in Dublin. Some of the distributors were concerned about the lead times for delivery for the first batches of R2-X. Reports from sales indicated that their phones were ringing off the hook from virtually every channel retailer across the globe. Malley painfully explained to them his inability to ship product until the end of the month. In the middle of his explanation, however, Malley was interrupted by a phone call deemed priority one. He excused himself politely and rushed to his office where he took the call.

"Ted. Randy."

"Great timing," said Malley. "Our friends in Dublin say advance orders are lighting up the switchboard. Europe is going nuts."

"Yes. I know."

"I told them they were clear for the 31st, but these guys are ready to play ball right now. And we're ready to go down here. Got rid of the generator glitches yesterday."

"Ted," Edmonds interrupted. His voice was controlled and deliberate.

"Yeah?"

"I want us to move into Phase II immediately."

"Are you serious? Now?"

"Crooks ran the numbers. It's the right thing to do."

"Six days?"

"Don't act so surprised, Ted. You've been in the industry long enough."

"That's only if there are no issues."

"Issues?" repeated Edmonds.

"Yeah. Only if our product is ready to go." Malley knew that in recent years, several large pharmaceutical companies had endured painful product liability lawsuits. Both Dow Chemical and Bristol Myers were virtually forced out of the market by a multi-billion dollar lawsuit concerning breast implant imperfections. Not long before, A.H. Robins was forced into closure by a similar lawsuit regarding the now infamous Dalkon Shield. Each case demonstrated that the product, despite passing federal requirements, had not been thoroughly tested.

"We're ready," Edmonds assured him. "Are you?"

"Two phone calls," answered Malley. "That's all it'll take."

"Good. Send out ten Selvas and begin production immediately."

"Ten?"

"That's right. Look. Nothing will hit the market until after approval but we need to move now. Let's build up some inventory. Stuff the channels."

There was a pause in Malley's voice. "We're jumping the gun."

"You are brilliant, Ted."

"What about the government down here, Randy?" Malley asked. "The leaks."

"You got enough man power for six days of production with our own people?"

"I suppose. Brazilian nationals don't report until the night of the 30th. They've completed their training. We were just waiting for you guys."

"Then this is an internal matter. Use only ex-pat staffing for these six days. If the nationals ask what you're doing, tell them this is a series of test runs before we can start and that we fully intend to honor our contractual agreements. You know the drill."

"You're the boss, Randy. But it sounds risky."

"I'm aware of the risks. What I need right now is someone I can trust down there. These six days mean light years down the road. As long as nothing ships until after the approval, we're fine. Let the inventory build up. Advance orders will easily deplete that by the end of the first week. And you'll be handsomely rewarded for your efforts."

"Okay, Randy. Ten Selvas?"

"That's right."

"You don't think the ICC will know? Sometimes they send reps down here."

"You're responsible for your own security at night."

"Yes."

"Have the trucks arrive at night then. In series of five if you can. It's only for six days. Hell, you're in the middle of the jungle down there."

"I'll do it, but-"

"It has to be done," Edmonds stressed. "I'm sure you understand."

Malley sat behind his desk with the phone dangling loosely in his hand. He didn't agree with Edmonds. Geniomics was asking for trouble in more ways than he cared to calculate.

PURSUIT

CHAPTER THIRTY-ONE

Hawthorn turned lightly beneath the covers as the bright morning sun cast glistening stripes across his bed. He sat up, rubbing his eyes, and then listened for the sounds of a faucet running in the bathroom or a cabinet being opened and closed. "Jordan?"

There was no answer.

"Jordan." She had already gone. This was her way of making a point. Damn her.

He winced at the thought of how he'd tell her about the trip. He could hardly believe what he was about to do. McAfee had already set up the meeting at Geniomics' R&D facility in Seattle for late in the afternoon. The men had met the night before for over five hours, going over and over the part he was to play. At least he didn't have to confront Williams again. He was scheduled off, even from ER, for the next two days. Jordan was going to freak. The timing couldn't be worse. Hawthorn flipped his legs over the edge the bed and traveled down the hall to the kitchen where Jordan, already dressed, was preparing to leave.

"I was about to wake you," she said.

"I thought you were gone."

"Soon enough."

Hawthorn opened the refrigerator and withdrew a half-filled container of orange juice. He reached into one of the cabinets to get a glass but could only find one clean candidate. The rest were piled high in the sink.

"We need to talk, John."

"You're right," Hawthorn answered. "You are absolutely right. Let's do it right now."

Jordan glanced over Hawthorn's shoulder to a clock on the microwave and laughed. "Nice. I can't. I'm already running late. Maybe when I get back. I'll be gone for two days, John."

"What? What do you mean two days?"

"Whatever. Don't act so surprised. I've told you this twice already. You're off in your own world expecting me to wait around for you. Negative, doctor. Now you can wait for me. I'll spend some time with someone interested."

"You going by yourself?"

"Yes."

"That's a long drive. What is it? Six hours to your Aunt's house?" She didn't answer him. Jordan was busy packing her cell phone into her purse. He was in the doghouse with a deadbolt fastening from the outside. "I'm concerned. That's all."

"Concerned? I've got news for you, John. The drive from San Jose to Portland wasn't exactly a cakewalk. And I did it when it was pouring. You didn't offer to come pick me up then, did you? Too busy."

"I don't know what to say, Jordan."

"That's the problem."

"Will you be okay?"

"Yes."

Hawthorn swallowed the last bit of orange juice and sat the glass lightly in the sink. "Well then, I've got some news for you."

"Great," Jordan said, rolling her eyes. She fastened the outside clasp on her purse and picked up her wallet in the other hand. She appeared determined to leave angry.

"I'm going out of town as well."

Jordan froze and looked at Hawthorn, astonished. "You have got to be kidding."

"Only for the night. There's a conference in Seattle the hospital is asking me to attend. I really don't have a choice in the matter."

"When?"

"What do you mean 'when'?

"When's the conference, John?" She stared at him with don't-BS-me eyes.

"Today."

"Are you serious?" Hawthorn shook his head. "And you're telling me now?"

"I'm sorry."

"Sorry? Sorry? Are you insane? I mean you can't be stupid or else you wouldn't be a doctor. What are you thinking, John? I haven't had a single second of your time. What in God's name are you thinking?" There were tears welling in her eyes.

"Jordan, please. I got in late. I just found out last night. Late."

"You amaze me, John. If you're going to be this inconsiderate- Screw it. I'm going with you. That's all there is to it." Jordan walked into the living room and headed straight towards the phone. "I'll just call Aunt M. and cancel."

"Jordan."

"I'm sure she'll understand."

"Jordan," he called louder.

"What?!"

"The hospital will only pay for one ticket. They only cover spouses."

"Money isn't an issue. This is ridiculous. How can they expect you to just drop what you're doing and leave? I'll charge it."

"Jordan. It's only for one night. The tickets cost five hundred bucks each. I'd much rather take you somewhere where we can relax and enjoy each other's company."

"John, can't you realize I've been trying to sit down and talk to you about-"

"Yes. I do," Hawthorn interrupted.

"Then why is it so damn hard to get a few moments of your time? This is crazy. I'm here for you. What is going on?"

"Jordan, something's going on at the hospital that…" He breathed deeply and looked heavily into her eyes, wondering if he should bring her into it. "Look, I know I've told you this before, but there's a lot of turmoil going on at the center and it's just not been a good time for me. I can't really discuss it right now because I don't have all of the answers, but it's very, very serious. When you get back, I promise the first thing I'll do is sit down with you and have this talk. Okay? I'm so sorry for these last few days. I really am."

Jordan opened her mouth to protest and then stopped. The look in her eyes told Hawthorn she finally understood something serious was happening. He held out his arms to gather her in as Jordan's face filled with concern. She wrapped her arms around him. "We need to talk, John. Things have got to change here. We can't go on like this."

"I know. I promise things will improve." Her kissed her on top of the head and then wondered if the words would ever find truth.

CHAPTER THIRTY-TWO

Hawthorn peered nervously through the plane's rectangular window, across a ruffled sheet of clouds. Far in the distance, above the delicate white blanket below, were giant pillar formations indicating a violent, westward-moving storm.

A flight attendant stopped by to see if Hawthorn cared for anything to drink. He declined. Hawthorn was already sick to his stomach with nerves and as far as he was concerned, nothing was going to make him feel better.

For the remaining fifteen minutes, Hawthorn studied his materials. He reviewed Geniomics' historical returns, their portfolio strategy, and the scheme to include their stock in a new biotech fund. When he finished, Hawthorn grabbed some identification cards and reviewed his personal information.

According to McAfee's plan, Hawthorn was scheduled for a tour of Geniomics' Research and Development facility in Bellevue around midday. He was to be received as Darren Bass, a financial analyst for the investment-banking firm of Hunter and Cox. McAfee had arranged for Hawthorn to sign a non-disclosure agreement and then be given access to select information so that he could judge the financial potential of several of Geniomics' future projects. This would allow him to get in, and get out.

Within minutes he was located in the back seat of a yellow cab, speeding quickly towards the Bellevue facility. He thumbed through the annual report and other information given to him the night before. There were awards, innovations and strategic relationships. The next time Hawthorn lifted his head, the cabby was pulling into the open parking lot of the Geniomics R&D stronghold.

"Mr. Bass. Mr. Bass," called a bald man, rushing out from the building's entrance. He was dressed in a white smock and held his identification badge in his right hand. "Good to see you. I'm Warren Dunn, the building coordinator here at the Bellevue facility. Glad you could make it. Please. Follow me. How long are you in town for?" he asked. Dunn flashed his badge to the building guard as both men passed through a metal detector.

"Just a day."

"Too bad," he said. "There's a double header against the Angels tonight. You should try and make it. Mariners may go all the way this year."

Dunn pressed his card to a badge reader on the wall, which opened the door to a facility conference room. After receiving a quick organization chart and corporate overview, Hawthorn was led to a small prep room. He was then instructed to step into a white jumpsuit that covered everything from his shoes up to his neck. Dunn handed him a white plastic hat that resembled a shower cap to cover his hair. "Right this way, Mr. Bass," he said, opening the door to the primary facility.

The interior was enormous. From his own estimate, he figured the length of the glass hallway to be close to seventy-five yards. Hundreds of research pods and cubicles lined the perimeter and were tucked neatly side by side between a thick glass barrier and the building's outside wall. According to a directory on a nearby wall, the main hallway wrapped itself like a glass tube around the building's center where most of the bacterial and infectious disease work was performed.

As Dunn pitched the promise of Geniomics' current and future projects, Hawthorn kept his eye on each and every visual clue. They passed a metal door under tight security that was labeled "Gene Therapy." Hawthorn had just encountered a recent article where Geniomics was praised for their efforts in developing a drug that could assist in regenerating the human spinal cord, a drug that held promise in helping to cure paralysis. On the next glass door, the painted words "Ocular Research" were covered with a hand written piece of paper that read "R2-X." A similar R2-X sign covered the next several areas as well. Obviously these workers were being redirected to work on the cold curing drug.

Dunn pointed through the glass wall at a researcher peering thoughtfully into his monitor's screen. "We have a state-of-the-art facility here in Bellevue, Mr. Bass. We offer a stable atmosphere for the brightest this world has to offer. And we are at the forefront of applying computer science to biology and chemistry innovations."

Hawthorn smiled and nodded his head. Stable? People were rushing from counter to counter, setting down and picking up vials of this and slides of that. Each time a worker exited or entered a new area, they would press their badge to a proximity reader, which would send a loud "beep" echoing through the lengthy glass hall. As these researchers continued to dart to and from their cubicles, chattering over the latest find, the narrow corridor was beginning to sound like a busy Vegas casino. Someone had set a fire beneath these people. The entire place appeared in a raving state of urgency.

Even the tour was rushed. The entire process lasted only one hour from start to finish and Hawthorn had yet to see or hear anything worthwhile. On the inside of the track were the protected labs and data center and on the outside were the office cubicles from which researchers, engineers, and managers could run computer simulations and conduct their private business. The only thing peculiar was the overwhelming amount of, what Hawthorn considered to be, "temporary" R2-X signs.

"How long has this facility been here?" Hawthorn asked, the hard soles of his shoes clapping against white tile. Another door opened and a set of four researches crossed the hall. *Beep.*

"It was built in 1990, so about seven years. We've expanded it several times, you know. Company's grown quite rapidly. We'll be doing it again, soon, I'm sure."

Hawthorn encountered another group of researchers eagerly working on cancer fighting bacteria. There were alternative forms of radiation and new types of antibiotics but nothing related to Mason's research. Even these areas had temporary R2-X signs.

Hawthorn asked on several occasions to see the interior portion of the facility. That's where it had to be. He'd seen everything else. Each time he was given an answer he felt was misleading.

"Very restricted access," he said. "Only a couple of labs like that in the country. Lots of bad stuff in there."

Hawthorn probably would have accepted it were it not for the fact that people were entering and leaving the central area with no special equipment or protective clothing. Why was he wearing a suit? There was nothing to indicate danger of any magnitude.

Halfway through the tour, Hawthorn broke free from Dunn's guidance and followed a researcher quickly into his nearby glass pod.

"Mr. Bass," Dunn called in an urgent tone. "Mr. Bass."

Hawthorn stuck his hand in the gap of the closing glass door to keep the lock from automatically shutting. A small magnet on the wall read: George Faldo.

"Excuse me, Mr. Faldo?" Hawthorn said, perched at the cubicle's entrance way. Faldo had already sat down and was punching the keyboard at record speed. "Excuse me. Sir?"

"Mr. Bass, I think we should let Mr. Faldo work."

Upon hearing Dunn's voice, Faldo immediately hit a hot key on his keyboard sending the computer screen into a sheet of black. He spun nervously around in his chair.

"Hi there. My name's Darren Bass," Hawthorn said, extending his hand. "I'm with the investment firm of Hunter and Cox in Portland. On a tour here." He could see Faldo's eyes float nervously between Hawthorn's visitor badge and Dunn standing behind him. "I was wondering if I could ask you a couple of questions."

Dunn reluctantly approved with a cautious nod.

Faldo was a heavier man whose large frame seemed incredibly ill-proportioned in his tiny, paper-filled cube.

"Just wanted to get a general idea of what types of projects you're working on here. You know. For the future. Of course, I'm under a full NDA, so your words are protected."

Faldo looked to Dunn for instructions who nodded a second time. "I assisted in the development of R2-X. Actually, I'm just now catching my breath from most of the testing. As far as the other projects go, I'm really not too involved there."

"What about neuro research? I hear it'll be one of the hottest fields in the next ten years. Another company we're considering is heavily involved there. We think it's going to be high growth."

"Yes," Dunn interrupted. He squeezed by Hawthorn and into the cube. "We've got a few projects involving the treatment of brain tumors and epilepsy but as far as I know, nothing is expected to be released until late '05."

"Nothing involving Alzheimer's?"

Dunn shook his head and smiled. "No. Nothing on Alzheimer's. Uh, Mr. Bass, that's all Mr. Faldo- That is all we are at liberty to comment on at this time. Geniomics makes it a point for each of the individual research teams to contain secrecy within their own groups until they are ready to go public with their findings. Frankly, I don't think anyone but the head of R&D really knows what's going on here at the fifty thousand foot level. Many of these ideas are still up for patent protection. Can't risk anything. Not even telling the researcher next door to you. Unfortunately there is no one here from upper management to answer your more technical questions accurately." Dunn patted Hawthorn on the shoulder indicating it was time to leave. "Thanks, George. If you'll excuse me, Mr. Bass, I have a meeting here in about 10 minutes, so I'll go ahead and show you to the dressing room."

As they walked the final leg towards the exit, Hawthorn could see the names of Geniomics' research management team posted outside of their office doors. He'd read the biographies of several executive staff members during the cab ride. Feldman. Gross. Binter. None of the names on the doors looked familiar until he got to the last one: Simon, Vice President of Research and Development.

As they passed his office, Hawthorn could see a young man sitting behind his desk toss up his hands while he talked on the phone. Dunn had lied.

"Well, thanks for coming Mr. Bass. I'm happy we had the opportunity to meet."

One of the large shipping doors in the back of the building slammed to the ground. As soon as it hit people started emerging from every cubicle traveling speedily towards the central area. Hawthorn stepped to the side as Dunn tried desperately to close the conversation.

"Thank you so much, again. And let us know if you need any further information." Dunn looked nervously over his shoulder towards the central area as two researchers strode past Hawthorn conversing back and forth over something Hawthorn could barely understand.

"This it?" one of the men asked.

"Yep, last one."

"Let's keep our fingers crossed."

Everyone was moving towards that area of the building. No one was wearing protective clothing. "What's all the commotion?" Hawthorn asked.

"Oh, it's nothing," Dunn answered nonchalantly. "We've been waiting on some field tests. Nothing too exciting. I really should be going to this little meeting, though. Just go through those doors right there and leave your suit in the white basket. The guard will let you out on the other side."

Dunn flashed his badge to the reader, which unlocked the door. "Take care now."

Hawthorn moved into the prep room and began to quietly disrobe, trying his best to gauge success or failure. Although he could sense something was amiss, Hawthorn was no closer to revealing anything that contradicted Mason's research. He was also no closer to exposing the tie that bound Geniomics and Dr. Williams. Aside from one dull conversation and an inadequate tour, Hawthorn didn't have a thing.

He stepped out of the jumpsuit and placed it neatly in the white basket. What now? Everything was a dead end. Hawthorn stared blankly at his image in the wall-sized mirror. He looked defeated. Maybe he didn't push hard enough.

As Hawthorn finished washing his face with two handfuls of luke-warm water, he noticed another door in the opposite corner of the room. He inspected the handle for a lock as he strode quietly across the tiled floor. It was open and, to his surprise, led back into the main facility.

Hawthorn peeked through the narrow gap. A few workers rushed towards the center of the building where the rest of the employees had gathered. The only thing separating them was the ID badge that hung from their necks on a small metal chain. Aside from that, many of the workers were either wearing their normal clothing or else white protective suits.

Hawthorn closed the door and quickly withdrew his white jumpsuit from the hamper. After he'd closed the final zipper and straps, he turned his visitor's badge inwards so that the only thing showing was the white backside of the card. He then reentered the now empty facility and moved stealthily down the glass corridor, encountering a few unsuspecting employees still straggling to the meeting. Each time they'd pass, he'd twist his body the other way as if he were looking for someone in one of the cubes. Hawthorn glanced through some large glass windows to the cancer center. Even they were gone.

After walking the perimeter of two more walls, Hawthorn located a researcher in the back of the building who'd remained to finish his work. The nameplate read: Ben Jenkins. He knocked gently on the cube's wall. "Excuse me."

Jenkins was a scraggly little man whose clothes looked many times too big for his frame. His proportions appeared locked into three parts brain and one part body as his large skull rested uncomfortably on a pencil thin neck. Jenkins was busy putting the casing on the back of his computer.

"Just let me get this thing." The casing snapped into place with a loud crack and he pressed a button to electronically unlock the large glass door. "You'd think they'd focus on quality one day."

"Can you tell me where the neuro area is? I just started a few days ago and I'm supposed to pick something up for Mr. Simon."

Jenkins gave him a funny look. "Neuro? That area was POSed three weeks ago."

"POSed?" repeated Hawthorn.

"Yeah. Put On Stop. Everything's practically stopped here. Everything except for R2-X. Hell, Simon knows that. He's the one that ordered it. Gotta get this stupid drug out the door. Wall Street's going nuts I hear."

"That's what I hear too." Hawthorn scanned his desktop for any clues. Nothing relevant that he could see.

"What's your name?" Jenkins was looking at Hawthorn's badge.

"Dan Wiley," Hawthorn answered, extending his hand. His ability to BS-on-the-fly was becoming automatic.

"What area you in?"

"Receiving for now. Maybe shipping in the next few weeks."

Jenkins nodded his head. "Great."

"I've seen the signs-"

"Yeah. Everything's R2-X. Hell, my project should be in the field right now but they cut me off. Bastards. Told me I had to POS it and help the clear the last hurdle. I said, 'Great. You want me to drop five years of work at the end of the cycle just to help the rest of these chimps get it out the door? I know it's a big one, but shit, do you really need the whole company to drop everything?' The ICC ain't going anywhere. But, you know. A job's a job. What the hell do we care? Just give me the damn paycheck, that's what I say."

Hawthorn nodded. "Me, too. What's going on over there?"

"What? Over there? Final tests I suppose."

"This late?"

Jenkins shrugged his shoulders and gave Hawthorn a funny look. "You never know."

Hawthorn flinched. Voices were pouring into the distant hallway. The meeting was over. Time to move. "Thanks, pal. Back to work."

"I'm not going anywhere," said Jenkins. Hawthorn was already making his way into the hall towards the prep room. "Just tell Simon to let me finish my project."

After narrowly escaping the view of several Geniomics researchers, Hawthorn arrived at the last straightaway that would take him to the prep room. Suddenly, he jerked back and paused at the hallway's corner. Dunn was talking to three other men just beyond the door. Hawthorn looked the other way. Two security guards strolled casually towards him.

Dunn didn't need the badge to identify him. He looked back towards the security officers. Thirty yards away. Surely they'd stop. He had to make a move.

Hawthorn jumped into the aisle and walked as calmly as possible towards the prep room door. Dunn was standing with his back to Hawthorn, yapping about something with the other three men. Hawthorn quickened his pace and then suddenly slowed twenty feet from the entryway. It was closed and needed a proximity reader.

Hawthorn looked behind. The two guards had already rounded the corner. He looked ahead. Dunn and the other men were shaking hands and finishing the conversation.

Hawthorn dropped to a knee pretending to tie his shoes. He undid his laces and then slowly tied them back together, praying the guards would pass him by.

"Okay, get those numbers to me soon," Dunn said, waving the other men off. He paused to write something down and then began to walk towards Hawthorn with his face buried in a notepad.

Just as Dunn and the guards were about to converge, another employee moved quickly past Hawthorn, pressing his card to the reader and opening the prep room door. Hawthorn lunged forward and followed quickly inside.

The door suddenly propped halfway open behind him. It was Dunn. "Sure. No. I don't mind at all… Of course." He was yelling something back towards the facility's interior with his leg and arm jammed inside the door.

Hawthorn yanked at the zipper. It was stuck. He pulled harder.

"Now? Can it wait? Jesus, all right." The door quietly closed as Dunn was called back into the main building. Ten minutes later Hawthorn was back in a cab headed for a Seattle suburb hotel.

CHAPTER THIRTY-THREE

Mason, meanwhile, endured yet another sleepless night. His entire evening had been spent on the hard wood floor of his living room, staring hopelessly at the hand-drawn map. For the past several hours, he'd battled the frightening sounds of desperate voices. Men and women alike. Screaming. Struggling. From time to time Mason could hear his mother's furious voice, howling as she pounded the blade into his father's chest.

Each time he would consume more pills from the unmarked bottle, although they no longer remedied the pain. This was how the night passed until at last, seated on the paper-ridden floor, the first rays of morning light cheated their way across the room.

Mason slumped at the edge of an antique chair, holding his map in one hand and a pistol in the other. In his lap was a swarm of individual bullets, each ready to be loaded into the revolver's bays.

He was a killer of innocent lives. There was no question about that. He could no longer trust himself. He'd become a tool for destruction. Mason removed the cap from the bottle and dumped an army of pills into his mouth, swallowing them whole.

BOOM. FLASH.

Mason found himself at a younger age, standing quietly outside his boyhood home. Behind him was the pothole-ridden driveway, leading from the roadway to a battered white home. Mason paused. Screaming voices emanated from inside the home. The young boy opened the screen door and quietly entered the living room. He peeked his head around the corner of the door.

"Understand? Understand what, Claire?" his father asked, throwing another glass into the wall. "I-"

Smash.

"Under-"

Smash.

"stand."

Mason bolted across the kitchen to wrap his arms around her but was greeted instead by the backside of his mother's knuckles. Mason was sent flying into the nearby garbage can. "Get out of here!"

"Goddamn't, woman. Keep your hands off him. Boy, go to your room."

Mason collected himself and walked back towards his mother. He was crying now. He held out his arms to hold her and again was sent plowing into the wall. "Leave us!" she yelled.

Mason hesitated. He wanted to help her. He wanted the fighting to stop.

"Get out of here, boy!" his father screamed.

Mason struggled to his feet and quickly left the kitchen. While the fighting continued, Mason went to his room where he laid on his bed, covering his ears and crying into his pillow. Each time he removed his hands from his head, he'd hear the sound of glass breaking or someone screaming at the top of their lungs.

After a while Mason spun his legs out of bed and walked the length of the hallway towards his parent's bedroom.

Mason dropped to his knees and reached far beneath his parent's bed frame. He pulled out an old-fashioned tobacco box and flipped open the lid. With shaking hands, Mason withdrew a small pistol. Just as he'd seen his father do on many a hunting trip, he opened the revolver and loaded one of the six chambers with a single bullet. When he finished, he took hold of the gun with both hands and headed back down the hallway towards the kitchen where the fighting continued.

"Enough," his mother yelled, holding a knife in her right hand.

"What are you gonna do with that? Put it down."

She shook her head. Her eyes were wild and she panted and heaved to catch her breath.

"There's no need for that, Claire. Put it down."

She refused to drop the weapon and started moving towards him.

"Put it down!" As he reached out to grab her, she swung hard cutting deeply into his arm.

Mason held his breath, his eyes wide with horror.

As she swung wildly again, his father fell backwards bringing the kitchen table down upon him. Overwhelmed with rage, she leapt onto his chest and lunged the blade deep within again and again.

"Momma, stop!" Mason shouted. He was eight feet away, pointing the gun loosely towards her head. His mother ignored him and continued to riddle his father's body with wounds.

Mason pulled the trigger.

Click.

"Stop," Mason cried, pulling the trigger again.

Click.

"You stupid man," she screamed thrusting the knife hard against his father's ribs. When her arms could give no more, she slid off his body and leaned heavily against the counter. Her blouse and pants were drenched with blood, and after smearing a streak of red across her face, she dropped the knife to the floor and let out a psychotic laugh.

Mason yanked the trigger a third time.

Click.

His mother picked up the knife and climbed to her feet.

BOOM.

Mason awoke from his vision still seated with the map in one hand and the pistol in the other. The pain and frustration was unbearable. He opened the six shot chamber and loaded one of the bullets. His mother's face had dark, evil eyes. Hate. And the blood. The terrible, terrible blood. Pools of it.

Mason raised the pistol to his face and placed the barrel softly in his mouth. He tightened his lips around the cold metal cylinder and closed his teary eyes.

"I love you," his mother whispered.

"No," sobbed Mason. "You lie."

The phone rang loudly from the kitchen. Mason thought of his patients; the young boy. Instantly, he pulled the trigger.

Click.

The phone rang again and Mason thought of Myra Floret. Twenty-three years old. It was his fault. A monster. Mason braced himself and screamed into the room.

Click.

He was feeling dizzy. He could see Mrs. Rose and her grandchildren. They were watching him. Laughing.

Click.

The barrel rattled against his teeth as tears flowed across his whiskered cheeks. He grabbed the pistol with two trembling hands and tilted his head against the wall, shoving the barrel deeper into his mouth. Mason coughed as his arms shook with anger and fear.

Click. Click.

The answering machine picked up. "Mason, please call me. I want to make sure you're okay. Please call me." It was Hawthorn.

Mason slowly removed the gun from his mouth and then angrily threw the pistol across the room. For the next few minutes, Mason cried. There was no way out. No way to back up and make things right.

Eventually, he gathered his belongings from the floor and retired to his bedroom where he would lay zombie-like for the rest of the day. For the next six hours he would endure the constant scream of his father's voice and visions of a blood-soaked blade.

CHAPTER THIRTY-FOUR

Hawthorn arrived at a Ramada Inn just outside Seattle around six o'clock that afternoon and, after battling through a lengthy registration, got on the phone and placed a call to McAfee. Since he was scheduled to return to Portland around ten the next morning, he wanted to make sure nothing had been overlooked.

"John. I was beginning to worry," said McAfee. "You're late."

Hawthorn stood at the window gazing tensely upon a Seattle suburb from his sixth floor window. The sky was clear with the exception of a few puffy clouds floating above the soft mango haze from the city's evening lights. "I know. I've been trying to sort this thing out."

"Well? How did it go?"

"That's what I'm wondering myself." Hawthorn pressed the phone to his ear with an arched shoulder and began thumbing through the Geniomics annual report that lay open on the small table. "Something's up there. No question."

"Yeah?"

"They wouldn't let me see much. It was a very fast tour. Very pushed."

"Doesn't surprise me."

"All they wanted to talk about was their cold drug. One guy said all other research had pretty much been put on hold till this one was out the door."

"Everything?"

"Apparently."

"Wow," he said. "That doesn't sound right."

"There was one area they wouldn't take me to. Said it was where they do their viral stuff. But something happened at the end of the tour and 'boom'- everyone left what they were doing to go there. I mean everyone. People from the cancer area, genetics, everyone. Completely unprotected. I don't know what type of research they're doing in there, but no one was wearing the protective clothing. And people were nervous. I mean, the looks on their faces said it all. And they told me there was no one from upper management there to answer questions- you know, when I started asking about the neuro stuff."

"And?"

"And on the way out I see the VP chatting on the phone in his office. Simon."

"Huh. Anything else?"

"That's about it. They said they had some neuro work going on, but nothing remotely close to Mason's. How about your end? Anything?"

"Haven't got the names yet. My contact's a little late, but I'm sure he'll have whatever is there for us. Shouldn't be long now. On another note. You gave a woman named Cindy my number."

"Yes," Hawthorn replied. "In case she needed to reach me. She's a contact at the center. I can't take any chances."

"Then you better call her. She found something, John. Something she said may open the door to this entire thing."

Hawthorn's next call was a page to Cindy who he knew would be at home early this evening. He keyed in the number to his hotel and the extension to his room and then hung up the receiver. Hawthorn desperately wanted to ask her what she new about this new drug. He hadn't thought of it before, but she'd mentioned long ago that she knew someone working in Geniomics' research division. Perhaps they could help shed some light on the situation.

Hawthorn slid around the edge of the bed and kicked off his shoes. His feet ached from the day's marathon. The muscles in his legs felt like they'd been separated from the bone. Hawthorn pushed himself across the bed and leaned wearily against the headboard.

He felt helpless. His day of fact-finding had gotten him nowhere. There was no evidence, no clues, and no one to talk to. The whole thing seemed too big for one person to tackle. Who was he kidding?

I'm a doctor for God's sake, he thought.

Why the hell was he tied up in all of this? He didn't ask for it. All he wanted to do was perform well and make his parents proud. Raise a family and live comfortably. Now look at him. He was in a no-win situation that was worsening with each passing minute. Trying to be a hero. For what?

Right now, all he had were his opinions. Even worse, Hawthorn realized that to bring this entire episode before anyone meant bringing it in front of the Center. Regardless of the outcome, he could kiss his career good-bye. The last thing he wanted to do was to ruin his career and let the real killer go free. He needed something solid. Something to fill the gaps.

Hawthorn picked up the remote control and flipped the it in his hands while he contemplated his position. Through the thin cracks beneath his doorway he could hear an older couple arguing over who was going to drive to dinner.

On the other hand, Hawthorn knew he was perhaps the only person who could expose what was going on here. The consequence of his inaction meant uncontested freedom for what could be a murderer of three. It could also mean the premature termination of a young physician's career who, perhaps more than anyone else in the world, had the potential to create value for all mankind. Then he thought of his father. Was it too late? He could hardly think about that. He had to pick the lesser of two evils:

look the other way and preserve his career or attack his suspicions and risk everything.

Hawthorn flipped to the Discovery channel. Two beetles appeared to be humping. He turned off the television. He was feeling sick with nerves. Jesus.

He had to keep going. Even if Mason was guilty. Not for his future or for his parents, but for himself. Here was a chance to do right. Regardless of the outcome or the risks involved, he had to press on. Hawthorn sprang from his bed, pacing back and forth across the room. He began to plot each event that had collectively resulted in his trip to Seattle. What he needed now, however, was information. Good, solid info.

The phone rang and Hawthorn quickly snatched up the receiver. It was Cindy. She was calling from a pay phone at a nearby convenience store. "Hawthorn. What are you doing in Seattle? You told me you were-"

"I know. I couldn't risk telling anybody."

"Well, I've got some information for you."

"Shoot."

"It's Benjamin, the janitor. Kerry found him with a pair of torn gloves stuffed in his pockets while he was cleaning the physician's lounge. Claims he got them in a wastebasket near 390. Mrs. Rose's room. I happened to have lunch with her right after. She'd just disposed of them so I snagged them."

Hawthorn's pulse quickened. "You have the gloves?"

"Yes." There was a slight pause. "And there's blood around a small tear."

"Blood? Was there blood found anywhere in the room?"

"No. From what I hear, no one found anything else."

"So what? So a doctor was busy doing something, forgot the procedure for exposure and left his gloves in the wastebasket. It may not mean anything."

"Well, that's what I thought at first."

"Wait, which glove is torn? Left or right." Hawthorn asked. Benjamin was left-handed. His right hand was maimed at birth.

"The left."

"And his hands?" Hawthorn had him. This wasn't the first time. Benjamin had been found alone inside of patients' rooms several times before.

"His hands are clean. And I can't take the gloves to the lab without logging them in the system."

"Jesus," said Hawthorn. He was staring out through his window at a sea of rolling hills and city lights. A DNA test would surely identify whose gloves those were. The administration kept detailed medical records on each staff member in case of blood contamination or some other emergency. "Don't tell me. Vinyl gloves?"

"That's the kicker," Cindy replied. "There were two layers of gloves on each hand. Latex beneath vinyl. The cut went all the way through. That probably explains why the police report you saw would have only detected vinyl. It was the only layer that touched everything. Latex would've never shown up. Unless it was from another doctor."

"Holy…" said Hawthorn. Mason was on the hospital's list of physicians who had to wear vinyl gloves. Any person naturally allergic to latex would suffer from a number of ailments.

It didn't make sense, though. Why would Mason go through the trouble of putting on an allergic, latex glove only to cover it with a vinyl one to which he openly subscribed? "The police report said there were vinyl prints all over the place, right? I mean those were the gloves that touched everything."

"Right. But there's more. 390's empty now so I went in there, unauthorized of course, and combed the place for any sign of blood or latex. Turns out we got the big one. Under one of the leg posts of the bed was a tiny piece of glove and some traces of blood. Looks like our mystery person dropped something and rushed to pick it up, tearing their hand on the bottom of the bed. Whoever it is has a deep cut on their hand. The piece matches the hole on the gloves exactly."

"Have you seen Briggs?"

"No."

"Williams?"

"No."

"What about Xiao?"

"Hawthorn, I just got out of that room a second ago. I haven't had time to look for anyone. You don't think any of them could have-"

"Who knows? A person who is normally allergic to latex gloves can easily wear vinyl ones with no adverse effects."

"Yeah," said Cindy. "But the only way a person would *need* to wear latex beneath the vinyl pair, is if…"

"… they want you to think they normally wear vinyl." finished Hawthorn.

"Should we go to the police? Obviously you don't want to go to Williams."

"No. Don't do anything until I get back. Just try to find the person with that laceration."

"I'll do my best."

"Good. Next, I need your help getting some information. What do you know about Geniomics' research?"

"They're in Bellevue."

"And?"

"Well, let's see. I have a couple of friends there from MIT working on some things. Haven't talked to them in a while, though. I think they're on the new cold remedy. R2-X they call it."

"They're working specifically on that project?"

"Yes, I believe so. One's a lead. Why?"

"That's all they're talking about up here. I really need to speak with someone close to the project."

"Wait a second, Hawthorn. We're friends, but I don't think they're going to risk their careers by giving you confidential information."

Hawthorn leaned forward at the window and gazed down upon the traffic six floors below. "We're at a dead end here, Cindy. We need another door."

After hearing his suspicions, Cindy reluctantly agreed to make the call. There was nothing in particular to look for, he explained, just any information that might lead to the next clue.

"I can't promise anything, Hawthorn, but I'll call them. They should be at home by now."

"Good. And don't forget to cover the Slyvy-M numbers for me," Hawthorn added. "You know where the key is."

Hawthorn immediately felt better. He was a step closer to identifying the killer but he still needed to expose the connection, if any, between Geniomics, Williams, and Mason. If he could find the killer perhaps that would reveal the connection. On the other hand, if he could find the connection, that could reveal the killer.

*   *   *   *   *   *   *   *

After surfing a few channels and dozing off for nearly three and a half hours Hawthorn awoke to find his head propped upright in the same position in which he had last been awake. Through squinting eyes, he looked at the message light on the phone. No one had called. The sleep felt great but now he was hungry. It'd been nearly fifteen hours since his last meal, a stale cherry bagel in Portland's airport. He picked up the phone and dialed room service but they were already closed. From the sixth floor Hawthorn could see a couple of fast food places across the street. He figured he could make it down there and back in five minutes. Just as he was about to leave the room, the phone rang.

"You're never going to believe this," said McAfee.

"Yeah?"

"I checked out the names, and it turns out the first two, uh... Kants and Bishops."

"Uh-huh."

"Clean as a whistle. Six bedroom house, successful, two point five kids, the whole bit."

"No records of any sort?"

"Nothing. They've each been with their corporation for over twenty years and they both have huge salaries. It'd be hard to find the motivation. I couldn't even find a speeding ticket."

"I suppose that's good."

Hawthorn slumped into a wooden chair at the table, browsing through the list of board members in the annual report. He read along as McAfee gave him their personal information. Halfway through the booklet he noticed a photograph of Geniomics' Board, each member standing in a thousand dollar suit with his arms glued to his side. He hadn't seen this before. Must have skipped right over it.

"Anyway," continued McAfee. "Who you'll want to hear about is Sam Mullin."

Hawthorn scanned the lines of the caption beneath the photograph with his finger. "I don't see him here. Nope. Sam Mullin is not in the picture."

"What are you looking at?"

"It's a group photo of Geniomics' board. Their annual report." Hawthorn flipped to the end of the manual to make sure he had given McAfee the right name. There it was. Sam Mullin. He flipped back to the photograph rechecking the names in the caption. He wasn't there.

"First of all, Hawthorn, you'll be surprised to hear that 'he' is actually a 'she'."

"Sam's a woman?"

"That's right."

There was only one woman in the photograph whose name was noted clearly below in the caption. "Then she's not here."

"Allow me to introduce you to Sam A. Mullin. Also known as Samantha Andrea Mullin. Maiden name… Williams."

"As in, Dr. Allen Williams?"

"Yep. Dr. Williams had a sister. Both were born to Gerard and Rebita Williams of Lexington, Kentucky. Their parents worked in the mines. Two children: Allen and Samantha. Both exceptionally gifted. There's your relationship. The weird thing was my contact came up empty on any other information."

"Like what?"

"Social security numbers. Medical records. Employment information. Everything was sealed. She's a ghost."

"Who sealed them?"

"Evidently someone pretty high up in the government. Not even my pals in DC could get into this stuff. Apparently the only thing available said Sam Mullin was deceased. No dates. Pretty weird, huh?"

"But she's listed here on their '96 board. Maybe there are a couple of them."

"Nope. He did find one article on Geniomics that listed her as an 18% owner but there was nothing else. He ran the check using a census database and then crosschecked that with every state d-base as well. She's the only one."

Hawthorn sat in silence trying to put this new piece of information into context.

"You still there?" McAfee asked.

"Yeah. Just thinking."

"About?"

"I was in Dr. William's office a few days ago and I saw this letter from him to someone named Edmonds. Edmonds, it turns out, is the CEO of Geniomics. It mentioned her name. It mentioned Sam."

"What was it about?" McAfee inquired.

"It had to do with offering Mason a huge research project. But the reference to her was almost personal, not related to the letter one bit. I can't really remember clearly but I can almost swear it referred to her as if she were alive. Jesus, I almost forgot I had seen that."

"So what we have here is a personal letter from Williams to the CEO of Geniomics talking about a research position for Mason. Why would Dr. Williams ever want to let Mason go? I mean, here you've got one of the smartest, most promising doctors on the globe from what I understand. How much were they planning on paying him?"

"A million a year," answered Hawthorn.

"Wow. They must really want him."

"See, that's the thing. They were adamant about having him start immediately, but what could he have done for them? Every resource they have is working on R2-X. Period. There's no reason to pressure him the way they were."

"Take a step back for a second, John. Look at what's going on here. First, you have Geniomics doing all that's possible to get Mason to drop everything and begin working for them immediately."

"Right."

"Then, you have a brilliant physician working on some valuable research for which he is about to gain substantial notoriety."

"Okay."

"And you would agree that Dr. Williams would never do anything to intentionally hurt his sister's significant position in Geniomics, correct? Assuming she's alive, of course. Eighteen percent is a huge position."

"I don't know their relationship, but yes, I would agree with that."

"The math is simple. One, Geniomics is going through a lot of trouble to lure a person who cannot immediately contribute. Two, you've told me Mason is working on some serious research and will be publishing his results soon. And three, we've agreed that Williams has a vested interest in the success of Geniomics. Add them up and I say that Geniomics and Williams want him immediately because he or his research represent a near term threat to R2-X."

"A threat?" Hawthorn asked. "A threat to what? His abilities are limitless. And he's a good human being. How in the world could he be a threat? Mason isn't working on the common cold, he's in neurology."

"What exactly was he working on?"

"A treatment for memory loss."

"And Geniomics is doing nothing else but R2-X?

Suddenly, Hawthorn's eyes grew to twice their size. "Jenkins."

"What?"

"Jenkins. A researcher at Geniomics. He said the ICC could wait. Yes. ICC. It makes perfect sense. The Conservation Consortium. Geniomics must need their approval, too. The meeting's two days away."

"Not sure I follow."

"The FDA won't consider their approval for R2-X final unless all of Geniomics' ingredients are affirmed.

Mason was to present his research there as well. It's the Goliath Zeteki-"

"Goliath what?"

"A species of frog. They're on the endangered species list. Mason needs access to its enzyme for his neuron-coating formula. Geniomics must need it as well. There's the connection. We got it." Hawthorn felt like yelling. "I'll be there in the morning, Doug. We got it. Pick me up at noon. We'll figure out what to do then."

Hawthorn hung up the phone and kicked off his shoes. For some reason he was no longer hungry. It was nearly one in the morning and he needed to get some sleep. He was getting much closer. He hadn't exposed the killer nor did he understand this Samantha Mullin character, but much needed information was beginning to make itself known.

RECKONING

CHAPTER THIRTY-FIVE

With a duffel bag draped around his shoulder, Hawthorn checked his watch as he entered a mirrored elevator that would drop him six floors to the hotel's ground floor.

"How can I help you, sir?" a bald man asked from behind the front desk. He wore a tidy blue uniform complete with red and yellow decorations on the lapel and shoulders.

"Checking out. 625," responded Hawthorn.

"I see. It'll be just a moment, Mr. Bass." The man disappeared through a doorway behind the counter and called out from the other side of the wall. "I'll just get you a print out so we can get you on your way."

Hawthorn's mind was ablaze with a game plan for the day. As far as he was concerned, his work in Seattle was finished. Now it was time to attack the issue at home.

"There you go, sir," said the hotel attendant, sliding the receipt across the counter. "Please come again."

Hawthorn smiled and signed his name across the bottom. He took his copy of the bill and stuffed it in the pocket of his jacket. A taxi was waiting outside.

"Mr. Bass," called the desk clerk.

Hawthorn stopped and turned.

A larger man emerged from the office in back. "Are you Mr. Bass? Mr. Darren Bass?"

Hawthorn glanced at the other man who showed no signs of surprise. He felt his stomach sink. "Yes?"

"There's a phone call for you. You can pick it up on that line over there," the man said, pointing to a phone mounted on the side of a wooden column.

"John. Thank goodness I caught you," said McAfee. "This stuff gets better and better."

"Go ahead."

"Last night, after we got off the phone. I was thinking about Samantha Mullin and why she would be deceased yet still listed on the board."

"Uh-huh."

"Remember how I said I'd done all the searches I could on the Board members and the officers? Especially Allen and his sister?"

"Yes."

"Well, as of yesterday I thought I had done everything I could. I mean, my man in D.C. had done every background check possible on Williams, Randy Edmonds, Samantha Mullin…"

"Ok."

"But it hit me that there was one avenue I had yet to explore: their parents. Turns out I was skimming through some Lexington Herald-Leader articles when I saw it."

"So, is she dead?"

"Just wait a minute. This is incredible. I ran into an article stating the adoption by the Williams family of an eight-year-old girl. Her real name is Gabriella Barcleaves. Apparently, Dr. Williams had a real sister named Samantha who passed away from some form of pneumonia when she was eight. From what I could gather Allen and his parents were devastated from the loss. There were subsequent articles saying how the courts were afraid to award them custody due to their apparent instability. Looks like our Williams had the hardest time of anyone. Apparently he never really accepted the new girl."

"Whoa," said Hawthorn.

"So I dug a little further to see if I could locate a Gabriella Barcleaves. There's a woman by this name in Castle Rock, just outside of Denver. Age matches exactly."

"Did you call her?"

"No. I wanted to give it to you. Maybe she can give us some information on Samantha Mullin. We've got to find out how this woman could possibly be listed as a member of the board when we know she doesn't exist. If Sam Mullin is truly deceased, we need to find out who controls her position. I'm sure Williams is connected."

"What should I ask her?"

"Who knows? She may not know anything. But I think you should call. We're running out of time and we still don't have all of the pieces. If you went to the authorities right now, what would you show them?"

"I'd show them Mason's serum."

"Fine. So you'd find a tie to Geniomics but what about Williams? And the killer?" Hawthorn had no answer. "We still don't know how Williams is connected in this whole mess. Maybe this Mrs. Barcleaves will help us."

"You're right. It can't hurt."

"Call me as soon as you talk to her. Here's her number."

"Okay. I'll let you know what happens right away."

Hawthorn hung up the phone and stared nervously at the paper in his hand. He glanced across the lobby and saw three phones located side by side on a short section of wall. They were divided by the men and women's restroom and seemed to provide adequate privacy.

Hawthorn moved into the corner phone and practically curled into a ball to shelter the conversation. As the earpiece clicked and clacked with the noises of a transferring call, Hawthorn spun a plastic calling card in his hand like a poker player down to his last trick.

The phone rang at least a dozen times. Just as Hawthorn was about to hang up, he heard the faint voice of an elderly woman. "Hello?"

"Hello. Mrs. Barcleaves?"

"Who is this?" she asked. The woman spoke with a Russian accent. "Why do you call here?"

"This is Darren Bass. I was hoping I could speak with you for just a moment."

"Gabriela is not able to speak with you right now."

"This is important. Please, it'll just take a moment."

"I said she is unable to speak with you right now. I take message for you."

"I just need a few seconds. I don't mean to intrude. It has to do with Samantha Mullin."

"Where did you hear that name?" she snapped. "Don't you ever quit? Let her have peace."

The woman hung up the phone and Hawthorn placed the receiver gently on the hook. He looked up and down the empty corridor. There was information to be had from talking to that woman. He glanced down at his watch: 8:03 a.m. His plane was to leave in one hour.

Hawthorn picked up the phone and placed another call.

"American Airlines. Can I help you?"

"Yes. I'd like to change a flight that I have leaving shortly for Portland, Oregon. Flight 1020 from Seattle. I need to go to Denver. But I need to be back in Portland by 5 p.m."

"I can get you back at 3:45. Although you'll only have a couple of hours in Denver."

"Perfect. That's all I need."

CHAPTER THIRTY-SIX

Mason's Bronco drifted its way down a worn asphalt two-lane that curved slowly back and forth like a snake through the northern Oregon forest. After passing through the small town of Scappoose, he snuck along a couple of back roads, over a small wooden bridge, and past a series of rural cabin homes tucked neatly away by the forest's edge.

As the road moved gracefully into a turn, his vehicle pulled slowly onto the shoulder and rolled to a halt. A badly weathered mailbox marked the beginning of a long dirt driveway that seemed to cut through a wall of pines. Way down, at the end of the quarter-mile drive, was a small abandoned home.

Mason stared at the broken house in the distance. He no longer fought the visions or dizziness. Instead, he searched each one for meaning; each dream dissected for the answer to what he felt was the intersection of his destiny and his past. Just as the dark spirit Bearcloud had invaded the life of Shepard Boone, so too had he found his way into the life of Mason Shane. There was no point in fighting it now.

Mason exited the vehicle and walked dazedly down the drive, each step bringing forth flashes of his boyhood existence. He could see himself racing to his bedroom after school, skipping and jumping across the puddles on his way down the drive. He could hear the echoing sounds of children's voices as they sang youthful rhymes from his childhood. Mason closed his eyes, taking in the soothing sounds of his childhood freedoms. It'd been every day of eighteen years since he'd been back.

Half way down the path, however, the voices changed. Replacing them were the frighteningly familiar sounds of two adults screaming and yelling at the top of their lungs.

Mason clenched his brow and glanced back down the road as if to consider leaving this horrible place. He looked at the house, its walls a collection of broken planks. There was no way he could leave. Not without finding her. He reached into his pocket and withdrew the bottle. There were only two left. His last chance to remember. His last chance to understand.

The many years of neglect had taken a cruel toll on Mason's childhood home. Many of the exterior planks had fallen to the ground and lay decaying at the base of the damaged building. Most of the windows had either been shattered by vagrant youths or destroyed by vicious winter storms. There were small mountain weeds exploding across the yard, each one puncturing the driveway's soil from the main road all the way to the front door.

Mason stopped short of the tiny porch that would lead him into the living room. He hated this place. He didn't need to go inside. This home brought nothing but anger at his life and despair with his family.

BOOM. FLASH.

The voices ceased as Mason found himself inside the home as a very young boy. He found himself walking calmly down the hallway from his parent's bedroom to the kitchen. He strode casually this time, floating across the hallway floor with a small handgun extending beyond his dangling arm. He moved past the living room and into the doorway of the kitchen where he stared emotionless at his father who whirled glasses across the room with all of his might.

Mason raised the gun and put his father in its sight. His mother had grabbed a knife. She was going to kill him. As she streaked across the room, Mason turned towards her

and pulled the trigger. Then he pulled it again. And again.
And again. And-

    BOOM.

    The front door slammed loudly behind Mason as he
moved into the sanctity of the living room walls. The warm
interior colors had long vanished and were now replaced
with pockets of dirt, broken floors, and thick layers of dust
covering everything in sight.

    A couple of chairs were stacked neatly in the corner
of the empty room beside a small bookcase where Mason
kept his texts for school. Beneath the chairs he could see a
small piece of paper that wriggled when the cold air blew in
from a nearby broken pane. Mason moved across the room
and lifted the paper in his hand. The document was barely
legible; the page's whiteness turned yellow with the passage
of time. He rotated it in his hands, examining its contents.
It was a grade report from his elementary school. It was the
first time he'd ever scored straight A's. He remembered
how rushed he was to get home and show his parents the
report. He'd entered the home that day with the piece of
paper locked tightly in hand.

    Mason crumpled the paper and tossed it to the
ground. He picked up a chair and launched it across the
room into an already broken mirror situated above the
fireplace. Fragments of glass flew in every direction.

    *"You don't give a crap about anything," Mason
could hear his father yell.*

    *"Calm down," cried his mother. "You don't
understand!"*

    Mason broke quickly into the kitchen and the voices
instantly disappeared. A stiff breeze howled past the jagged
glass of another broken window causing the cupboard doors
to swing from side to side.

    Across the dust-covered tile, Mason could see the
table that his father had pulled down in his last breaths of
life. It had remained on its side as he'd seen it on that

fateful day. His father had gasped for breath when she'd stuck him the very first time. He remembered how his limbs flailed in every direction as she sliced him on the ground.

Mason left the kitchen and walked towards his parent's bedroom, careful to avoid oblong holes riddling the hallway floor. All in all, it looked as he remembered. His parents' sheetless bed remained situated beneath a large window in the middle of the shattered room. The dresser, although badly collapsed, was located in the same corner as he remembered and the door to the bathroom, though broken badly, sat neatly propped up against the doorjamb.

Mason flicked on the lights. No power. He moved around the edge of the bed towards the dresser, watchful of the broken beams prodding up from another hole in the floor.

The bed creaked loudly as the springs beneath the mattress sounded their surprise to a familiar guest. Mason looked over the dresser's six drawers, one of which was missing a handle. His mother had ripped it off when the police came to take her away.

The howling wind outside of the room's only window caught Mason's attention. He looked up at the weathered strips of curtain hanging at the window's edge. They appeared as if they could crumple with the slightest touch. Mason stared at his reflection in the dresser's broken mirror. He barely recognized himself. He'd been given such a miserable life. He reached forward to one of the drawers and pulled it open.

Mason propelled backwards across the bed. The drawer was filled with insects that jumped onto the mattress and floor. He yanked a splintered board from the floor and forced himself against the far wall as the sea of bugs quickly covered the decaying mattress and floor. Mason turned for hallway and then wrenched his body backwards against another wall. His mother stood naked in the doorjamb with a knife in her bloodied right hand. Her eyes were colorless beads and thick sets of lacerations formed burn marks around the base of her neck.

"Mason," she called.

"I hate you!" Mason yelled, swinging wildly at her body. The board smashed against the edge of the doorway and splintered into pieces.

"Mason," he could hear her say. Her ghostly figure now stood just inside the kitchen at the far end of the hall.

Mason grabbed the broken end of the board and launched himself into the hallway. She would pay for what she'd done. As Mason raged towards the kitchen, drops of blood dripped from the force at which his hand clenched the splintered board. His face was tense with fury and as he rapidly hopped and danced over the holes in the hallway floor, he gathered a tremendous speed.

Mason burst into the kitchen, throwing the board angrily against one of the broken windows. As his feet slid from beneath his body, Mason threw out his arms to cushion his collision with a wall of cabinets. Doors and shelves flew in every direction as he slammed hard against the wall and fell to the tiled floor. Fifteen feet away, his mother was sitting upright on top of his father's bloodied corpse. The pool of blood was enormous and moving his way. His father was looking with open eyes to Mason for help. Mason coughed and gagged. His father's chest was pocketed with an uncountable number of wounds.

Mason scrambled backwards and crashed heavily into the damaged table. In an instant, the figures were gone. Small drops of water fell next to him on the kitchen tile.

Slowly, Mason rose to his feet as he gathered in the true state of his surroundings. His pants were drenched in water and he struggled to regain his breath. He wanted to kill her. He wanted to rip out her eyes and slice through the bones in the back of her neck.

Mason placed his hands on the edge of the sink and peered through a window towards his car at the end of the road. He wouldn't stop until he found her. She was not out of his life as he'd previously thought. There was work to be done. So be it.

Mason coughed and spat into the rusted sink. Suddenly, his brow angled with understanding. The visions and dreams, this map and note, were finally making sense. They would bring him to her. He would see for himself. Mason regained his composure and left the small white house. He couldn't wait to find her.

CHAPTER THIRTY-SEVEN

Hawthorn's flight from Seattle to Denver was marked by turbulent bumps and sweeping skids that tossed the large plane from side to side like a twisting roller coaster, a buffeting movement that seemed to mimic his emotions.

As his cab rolled through a wealthier part of Denver, Hawthorn found himself glued to the window, gazing at the spectacular homes that dotted the tree-covered hillside. The Barcleaves' estate must be enormous, he thought. The lot sizes alone were doubling every five houses.

The large mansions, however, soon turned to middle class homes. Moments later these too disappeared, giving way to lower-income, publicly funded housing projects. Hawthorn looked at some weathered numbers on the buildings as the cab cruised past. They were getting close. Two minutes later, the cab pulled along side a foot high curb just outside a small, beige-colored home.

"This is it," announced the fat cabby. "That'll be thirty-three flat."

Hawthorn withdrew the small slip of paper and double-checked the address against a set of rusted numbers hanging loosely above the front door. This was it.

The small beige home left much to be desired. The sidewalk beneath his feet appeared badly damaged from years of neglect. The city of Denver obviously didn't pay much attention to this side of town. The house looked even worse. It wasn't an ugly home. One could tell it was once a charming little abode, perfect for a small, middle class family. Its decay was no doubt marked by some other event. Perhaps the town grew in another direction and the neighborhood lost its charm.

The yard was yellow and uncut and outlined by a chain-link fence with holes and broken links in almost every measure. Hundreds of weeds surfaced from the ground, disrupting the even flow of what must have once been beautiful natural turf. No one had cared for this place in quite some time.

A brisk wind blew open an old newspaper on the front porch as Hawthorn moved slowly through a waist-high gate that squeaked when it opened and clanked loudly when it closed. Two wooden steps elevated him to the main porch. He pulled his jacket in close around his neck and gave three light raps on the decaying screen door.

At the end of the porch was an old-fashioned pail placed perfectly beneath a broken gutter. It didn't make sense. Adopted or not, how could Williams' let his own sister live like this? Eighteen percent? Hawthorn knocked again, this time a little louder. Someone was playing with the chains and locks on the other side.

The door slowly cracked open and then stopped, still connected by a single metal chain. Through the thin opening Hawthorn could see the wrinkled face of an elderly woman staring at him with a nervous, fidgeting glare.

"Yes?" She appeared ready to slam the door.

"Mrs. Barcleaves?"

"What business you have here?" the woman asked. "What do you want?"

"Hello, ma'am," said Hawthorn, speaking as pleasantly as he could. "I was hoping I could speak with Mrs. Barcleaves."

"She's not here," responded the old woman.

"Do you know when she might return?"

"Not for long time." She was already closing the door. "Now thank you for your time."

Hawthorn opened the screen door and put his hand in the doorway. "Ma'am, I don't mean to bother you, but I've come a very long way just to say hello. I'm the son of one of her very good friends from Lexington." The woman's face lightened and expressed a sudden interest. "My mother passed away a month ago and she asked me to see Gabriella."

Hawthorn rubbed his hands together pretending to be cold. "I'd just like to see her. I won't stay very long."

"What is your name?" she asked.

"John Hawthorn. My mother's name is Rue."

The woman looked him over with probing eyes and then slowly closed the door. Hawthorn grimaced and then looked out at the street. He'd blown it. Rue? Of course she wouldn't buy it. He hated to lie but he had to talk to her, even if only for a moment. He glanced back to the closed door wondering what the hell he was going to do next. A few seconds later the final chain was undone and the door opened.

Walking into the main living room was like stepping back in time. It was small and boxy with thick green curtains and a dull wooden floor. The furniture was old, perhaps from the turn of the century, and covered with multi-colored, Afghan quilts. Stacks of old newspapers and hardcover books were piled on every surface. Hawthorn could see a rotary phone but other than that there were no signs of modern electronics.

Black and white photographs embellished the mantle above the fireplace. Hawthorn could see an 8 x 10 photo of Gabriella and Allen as small children. His father was holding Allen charmingly while the similar aged Gabriella stood off to the side somewhat discontent.

"Please, have a seat," the Russian woman said as she disappeared into the kitchen. "Can I get you something to drink? Tea, perhaps?"

"Please. That would be great," Hawthorn answered. It'd allow him to stay longer.

"Tell me your mother's name again." The old woman returned with two cups of tea on a platter. She rested her own cup on a small coaster as she eased carefully into the lap of a worn, tub-styled chair. "When did she know Gabriella? Must have been some time."

"I'm not really sure. I suppose when they were very young. It was quite a surprise when she me gave Gabriella's name. Is she here?"

The old woman nodded. "She's here."

"Will I have the chance to see her?" Hawthorn asked politely.

The woman raised her hand telling Hawthorn to wait while she sipped another drink. Hawthorn glanced at the grandfather clock in the corner of the room. He had slightly more than an hour before he'd have to get back to the airport.

"First about you," she said. "Where are you from?"

"Texas. Austin to be exact. Mother loved the hill country. Wanted to be somewhere beautiful when she passed."

"And what do you do there?"

"I'm a financial planner. It pays the bills."

"And what you know about Gabriella, Mr. Hawthorn?"

He looked curiously at the doorway leading to the kitchen. Gabriella had yet to surface. He listened carefully for any noises coming from the distant corners of the house but there was nothing. The only sounds breaking the deadness of the house were the old woman's tongue and the methodical tick-tock of the grandfather clock.

"I know she was born alongside my mother in Lexington around 1932 and that she had a brother named Allen. I know her mother and father worked in the mines and that her father eventually passed away when he was about thirty-four or so. Black lung, I hear."

"And why you suppose your mother sent you here?" she asked intently.

"I believe she felt Mrs. Barcleaves-"

"*Ms*. Barcleaves," the woman corrected him.

"Ms.?"

She nodded her head. "Gabriela married for only a few months. She was twenty. Her husband was ill. Died before she could help. She never remarried."

"Never?"

The woman looked firmly into Hawthorn's eyes like a mother about to tell a child some very bad news. She then returned her cup to its coaster and stood from her chair. "Follow me, Mr. Hawthorn," she said. "I will take you to Gabriella."

Hawthorn followed the old woman out of the living room and down a long and narrow hallway that led to the back of the house. When the passage came to an end, the two ascended a tri-level, quick turning staircase that lead to the second story of the aged home.

The upstairs hallway was also dark and contained no doors except for one leading to a brightly lit chamber at the very end. Soon enough, the dark wood panels gave way to a sunlit room with bright yellow walls and a freshly polished floor. Just outside the door, the Russian woman paused and took Hawthorn by the arm. "I'm sure she'll be happy you were able to stop by. She rarely has visitors these days."

Hawthorn smiled uncertainly and nodded his head. There was something in her voice. Rarely has visitors?

As the two entered the room, Hawthorn's jaw dropped open with amazement. There were flowers everywhere. Every color of the rainbow seemed represented: roses, violets, tulips, lilies, and orchids. Sunlight beamed in through a wall of glass windows, ricocheting off the polished wood floors.

As the woman lead him further into the room, Hawthorn's smile slowly disappeared. The sounds he was hearing from around the corner were all too familiar.

Tucked comfortably beneath some plain white sheets, amidst the colorful flowers, was Gabriella Barcleaves. To her left was a pulse monitor. To her right, an IV tower. And behind her head, the respirator which allowed her to breathe.

Gabriella was a frail woman whose face displayed the psychological wear of a much older person. Long, free-flowing silver hair extended beyond the pillow only to disappear through a gap between the bed and the respirator machine. There were no wrinkles in the sheets. Hawthorn could tell she'd been laying in this position for quite some time.

"Look, Ms.-"

"Kropov," the old woman answered. "I've lived with Gabriella for many, many years. We are best of friends."

"I'm sorry," he said somberly. "I didn't expect this. I don't know what to say."

Hawthorn stared at Gabriella and pointed to her as if to ask whether Gabriella could hear them.

"Mr. Hawthorn," she said. "Gabriella Barcleaves has been in a coma for nearly ten years."

Hawthorn swallowed heavily. Her face wore a peaceful but sad facade. It was hard to imagine she could be related to a someone like Allen Williams. A clock on a nearby dresser indicated he had less than forty-five minutes to get back to the airport. Time was running short.

"Mrs. Kropov," Hawthorn said apologetically. "I need to admit something to you. I'm not a financial planner from Texas. In fact-"

"Of course you're not," she said. "On the contrary, I'm sure that you come for other reason. I can see it in your eyes. They are sincere."

"Thank you. I'm sorry. I need to know what you can tell me about Samantha Mullin."

"Where did you hear that name, Mr. Hawthorn?"

"I-"

"You are never to repeat that name in this house again. Is that understood? That name brings nothing but pain to Gabriella and everything she once believed in. I don't know how familiar you are with Gabby's life, but it has been one of misery. This world has placed Gabby at the mercy of monsters."

"Like her brother Allen."

"So you know of her brother."

"Mrs. Kropov, I've come here today from Oregon because I am a doctor who works with Allen Williams in Portland. And I have strong suspicions that he is involved in some very controversial matters."

"Not surprising."

"I know that Allen had a younger sister by the name Samantha. I also know that Gabriella was later adopted when Samantha died and that she probably endured some serious trauma."

"You don't know half of it. Samantha was born a year before Allen. Samantha got sick. The doctors thought it was a virus but rumors persisted that Allen had given her a cleaning chemical to help cure her of the flu. He loved her but ultimately *he* was the one responsible for her death. I am told he would go for four or five days without sleep while he sat next to her bed watching her die."

The woman walked over to an old dresser where she removed a necklace from around her neck. At the end of the chain was a small key that she used to unlock the top drawer.

"Allen was eight when this happened?" Hawthorn asked.

"Yes." She withdrew an old scrapbook that she opened on the top of the dresser. After flipping past a few pages, she motioned for Hawthorn to stand beside her. "These are articles from that year. Gabriella got them from the city library in Lexington. See?"

The open page highlighted five articles. Three discussed the mysterious death of young Samantha and contained multiple quotes from baffled physicians. The next was an interview with the distraught parents and the next probed boldly into the possibility of foul play.

"They say that was when he decided to be a doctor. He could not live with the pain. Guilt is more like it."

She flipped forward to another article, which showed Dr. Williams in high school. He was questioned for a minor explosion in the chemical department. Two others showed him being interrogated for stealing some animals from the biology labs in college. Hawthorn paused. The last article was dated twenty years ago. Williams claimed he was close to finding a cure for the common cold.

"So Allen's parents adopted Gabriella shortly after Samantha died?" Hawthorn asked.

"Immediately. She was abandoned in the forest when she was an infant. Allen had a difficult time adjusting. He refused to call Gabriella by her name and would only refer to her as Samantha. You can imagine what that would do to a young child. For years this went on. The torture."

"And the parents?"

"They cared for her until the father got sick. Gabriella told me as much as she could remember, although her memory did not recall much. Who could blame her? The mother turned her attention from the children to care for the husband. Allen would lock her in the closet for a full day and night until she'd answer him as that name. She told me he would play these games with her every moment he could. Many years later, he made her change her name legally to Samantha."

"And the name Mullin? That was from her husband?"

The woman nodded. "You can see why those names would hurt her so."

"She never remarried?" Hawthorn asked delicately. He could tell by her features that Gabriella had once been a very attractive woman.

"Allen wouldn't allow it. He controlled everything, that man. Each time she would get involved with someone, he would make it miserable for everyone. Extremely jealous. He kept a very tight grip on her." The woman placed the scrapbook in the drawer and locked it with her key. She then tucked the necklace safely beneath her blouse. "All her life, Gabby has been reminded of how the Williams' saved her life. Allen never let her forget it."

The woman then lowered her voice. "Then, about fifteen years ago, Allen quit bothering her. Stopped the calling, the unannounced visits, everything. Every once in a while he would call but for the most part, no contact. We thought he was finally ready to let go."

"And?"

"Five years later, Gabriella came down with a very bad cold. It later turned to pneumonia. The physicians told her that if she took the medication she would recover. You see, she moved here because she wanted to get away from him."

Hawthorn nodded.

The older woman continued, "Allen found out about her sickness and rushed home right away. He'd been working on some private research with another corporation. An advisor, I think. He was very worried that day, not like the times before."

"This is ten years ago?" Hawthorn clarified.

"Yes. Gabriella is in trouble with her health. She was sick. And alone. Allen talked her into surrendering control of her treatment to him. She signed many documents. He would put them in front of her and she would sign."

Hawthorn figured she'd been poor for several years and most certainly would never have been able to afford quality care.

"Allen changed her medication. Said everything would be all right. She did what he said and that's when it happened."

"What?"

"She fell asleep never to wake up again."

"A reaction to the medication."

"I am sure of that."

"And did you tell you anyone?" Hawthorn's heart ached for what Gabriella must have endured.

"Yes. The state wished to place her in a low-cost retirement home. I could not allow that. I could not afford a lawyer. I contacted the public defender's office who contacted Dr. Williams."

"And?"

"And Allen claimed he'd done nothing wrong. That he had given her the standard treatment. Somehow, he had all of the documentation to prove it. He offered attorney the opportunity to win the case since he would pay for all of the necessary hospital equipment to be placed here in this home. We were told it was our best alternative unless we could come up with insurance."

Hawthorn was speechless. No words could be found to lessen the pain and frustration these women had endured.

"What kind of trouble is Allen in now?" Ms. Kropov asked.

"He may be tampering with patients. It may involve murder. I mean, I don't know whether or not he did it, but he's definitely involved."

Ms. Kropov left the dresser's side and walked into a small closet where she yanked on a cord to turn on the light. "You are a doctor, correct?"

It sounded as if she were pulling something off one of the top shelves.

"I would like to show you something. Perhaps you can make sense. I managed to hide one in this box." She emerged from the small walk-in with a shoebox covered in dust. "I don't know what it means- if anything."

Kropov placed it gently on the top of the dresser and carefully removed some worn tape that had held the lid tight for several years.

Hawthorn could see a small roll of paper placed neatly among the other trinkets. She withdrew the papered coil and carefully unwrapped a small prescription bottle.

"This is one of the medicines Allen gave to her ten years ago."

Hawthorn spun the tinted bottle in his hand. It was clearly a homemade concoction from William's own library of experiments. As a novice chemist, he'd labeled the drug a "controlling device for the common cold." And his own sister, the guinea pig.

The bottle also explained Williams' interest in Geniomics' cure for the common cold. On the very bottom he could see the faint markings of a long since extinct Geniomics logo. Williams must have tried his best to perfect the formula alone, and when he could go no further, he sought out a young entrepreneur with the missing link.

Hawthorn thought about Williams' arrangement with the Center. The problem must have been that he was legally unable to put his own money into the company without surrendering his job at the CME, a role he cherished more than life itself. Hawthorn knew that the top two positions at the hospital were prohibited from investing in any type of biotech company for this very reason. In a way, Williams probably felt that this was his project to be had. The money resulting from the cure was to be his. *He* wanted to be the one to cure the world and his sister was the perfect funnel for ownership. There were no records, no one knew her, and she wasn't going to talk to anyone for a long, long time.

Hawthorn figured Williams would be the primary beneficiary of her stock position. That meant that the assets would pass to him only when she died. Since his present contract with the CME wouldn't allow him to take it a moment earlier, he had to keep her alive until he fulfilled his work contract. With that amount of stock, he stood to make millions. If R2-X was a hit, that number would grow tenfold.

A few minutes later, Hawthorn hugged the old woman good-bye and promised to do everything possible to bring Allen Williams to justice. The last piece to the puzzle was to expose the killer. Clearly, Williams had motive. If he had a laceration on his left hand, Hawthorn had his man.

CHAPTER THIRTY-EIGHT

Randy Edmonds sat proudly at the far end of a sleek, ebony conference table in Geniomics' executive boardroom. He'd adorned the War Room, as it was called, in every last bit of modern technology: self-adjusting networked chairs, teleconferencing, remote lighting, and high definition plasma collaboration screens.

Stationed around the perimeter of the oval table were the top three executives from each functional discipline: Marketing, Finance, Operations, and R&D. With the ICC approval hearing only one day away, the purpose of this meeting was to square away the final operational details before the official public release.

Earlier in the day, Edmonds received an updated report showing each of the international business units' projected demand for the next fifteen months. These numbers were based on advanced retail orders from resellers planning to stock the drug for consumer use. He'd prepared several slides to communicate this to his top men.

"Gentlemen, the time has come to quit reading about history and start making it. I've received new demand reports indicating R2-X will far surpass our original estimates."

The lights lowered as the wall behind him filled with a backlit presentation slide entitled "No Limits." Edmonds paced around the oval table as each member of the executive team gazed over the material.

"Europe is responding overwhelmingly. Pre-sales are exploding all previous records. It appears we are truly at a crossroads for a new generation of medicine. I've received a report stating that demand for R2-X right here in our own backyard may approach twice the original forecast."

There was excitement as the other executives commented to each other in confident whispers. Edmonds paused at the opposite end of the table, staring past each of his men to the brightly lit screen in the background. "What I want to know is if we will have the necessary resources to fill this demand. I'm aware that we'll have a significant level of backlog for some time but I want none of our demand to transfer to the competition. Am I clear? Bottom line. Can we produce this stuff quick enough?"

"Yes, Randy. Ted's confirmed there's enough resources in the South American operation to fuel the initial peak. Operations should not be a problem."

"Fine," Edmonds said. "Folks, as you know, we're planning to attend ICC hearing tomorrow. I expect everything to proceed as planned with the FDA granting their approval shortly thereafter. Is there anything we may have overlooked?"

Ken Camden from Marketing nervously tapped his pencil and turned the question towards Research. "Simon," he said. "Are the test results documented and ready to go?"

Simon nodded. "Yep. Right here." He withdrew a large binder documenting each of the tests that the ICC and the FDA would need to see before granting their final approval.

Camden then shot Edmonds a deliberate look, letting him know he wasn't thrilled about what they were going to do.

"And the marketing collateral is distributed?" Edmonds asked. "How about you, Ken. You ready?"

"Everyone's prepared," Camden answered, purposefully short.

"Is there something wrong, Ken?" Edmonds asked. "Need I remind you that you will be a multi-millionaire after this is over?"

The group chuckled as Camden faked a humble smile. "No, Randy."

Edmonds strolled to the other end of the long table as the screen changed to the next slide. "Good, because *we* are making history. No one has ever discovered and brought a drug to market faster than this team. No one has blended technology and medicine like this team. Your efforts will bring to bear the new dawn of intelligent medicine; drugs that can cure, adjust to a changing environment, and continue to cure based uniquely on the genetic make-up of the host."

Edmonds paused, letting his men feed on the energy of the moment. Then he lowered his voice.

"Never in the history of mankind have we been able to permanently suppress the simple common cold. This company and your hard work will change that. I thank you for being part of this adventure and I challenge you to work even harder. This company prides itself on operational excellence. We are biological technologists. Let us never forget that. What time are we to meet in San Francisco tomorrow?" He was talking to his executive assistant.

"Hyatt Regency at nine. Hearing at one."

"For those of you attending with myself, Geniomics One will leave at 6:45 this evening. Once again, thank you very much for everything you do. Lives across the world will be grateful as well."

The lights quickly returned to normal as each of the managers gathered their notes. Edmonds shook a few hands and then quickly made his way to Camden.

"Ken, would you like to talk about this?" he asked quietly. "I know what you're thinking and I can identify with that. But, aside from the money, there will be much more good done here than bad. Do you understand? You are going to be rich. Filthy rich."

Edmonds slapped him on the back and exited the room.

CHAPTER THIRTY-NINE

Hawthorn arrived at gate 14 inside Denver's tent-shaped airport with only five minutes to spare. A digital display behind the booth indicated that flight 455, inbound from Chicago O'Hare, would be delayed for another hour. Apparently there was a bad fog in the Chicago area delaying most of the afternoon's flights.

Hawthorn quickly located another wall of phones. It was time to come clean and tell Jordan everything. He'd kept her in the dark long enough. There was no way he could accomplish what he needed to without telling her what was going on. Hawthorn waited painfully through the rings and then his own voice on the machine. There were two messages.

The first was from Jordan. "John, it's about twelve thirty and I'm running late. They've planned a surprise party here for me so I'm going to stay and eat lunch with them. I don't know when exactly I'll catch you, but I'm looking forward to talking to you later this afternoon. Bye."

Hawthorn stood with his back to the base of the phone, gazing across the sea of people. There was a couple in the distance holding hands.

"Hawthorn. Cindy. Uh, I'm sorry to bother you at home, but I think you should contact me soon. You'll want the lab results on those tests you were looking for."

Hawthorn could hardly fathom what she may have uncovered. As he hung up the phone, a commotion broke out on the other side of the building. A couple of boys had tried to make off with someone's luggage and were caught by airport security. He felt like telling them to let the kids go. After all, what was stealing a bag of luggage when compared to putting your sister in a coma?

Hawthorn considered calling Mason. He reflected on the last time they'd spoken. The middle of the cemetery. "Shepard Boone," he remembered. And Bearcloud. The picture in the cafe. The Grizzly bear and the angry man with the scepter. Impossible.

With a sick feeling in his stomach, Hawthorn returned Cindy's call.

"Get ready for this," she said, half out of breath. "I just got off the phone with my friends in Geniomics- I told them everything. They're changing trial results, Hawthorn. One of them saw a note from the head of R&D to the president. A lot of people could get sick from this. They're planning to lie."

"Will they help?"

"They'll help if we can prove a link to these murders. They're scared, John. They don't know what to do."

"Geniomics needs the enzyme."

"Yes, I know."

"What about the glove?" Hawthorn asked. "Anything?"

To her dismay, most of the usual suspects were completely clear. Williams was gone for the afternoon. Xiao was scheduled to be in meetings most of the day, but the admin in Pathology said she hadn't noticed any injury to his hands when she'd spoken with him that morning. Brenner was clean, as was Dr. Howard, Dr. Clark, and Dr. Outland.

The only real news came from Briggs. He'd exited the surgeon's washroom with his left hand forged deeply in his pocket. Cindy then followed him secretly through the third floor, past the nurses' station, and into the elevator. At first she thought nothing of it but as the minutes progressed, she noticed that he still hadn't withdrawn his hand. Eventually, he went into William's office and never came out.

"I knew it," said Hawthorn.

"That's what I thought, too. Until I ran into Rector."

"Rector?"

"Yeah. I was down near forensics getting a signature." She went on to explain how she'd spilled ink on her smock. She stopped in a small janitorial lavatory to wash up before going back up to the lab. As she scrubbed her hands, the door opened and Rector slipped inside.

"I was scared," Cindy recalled. "I could hardly speak. The room was barely big enough for three or four people."

"Cindy. What brings you down here?" Rector asked.

Cindy immediately looked for his left hand, now tucked away in a coat pocket. "Getting a signature, Dr. Rector. Excuse me."

As she moved past, Rector leaned in close and whispered, "Listen to me. Be careful, Cindy. The two of you are messing with people way out of your league."

"So I remained silent. I was too frightened to move," Cindy explained. "'Just know,' and for this he lowered his voice and pointed in the air, 'they're always watching us.'"

Hawthorn was stunned. "He's involved."

"Now wait a minute, John. Draw your own conclusions if you want but that doesn't necessarily mean anything. But he, and someone else, knows we're looking."

"I completely overlooked it- Rector's the next one to take command. He's waited his entire life for this. If Williams could get anyone to do it, it's Rector."

"You may be right, but that's assuming quite a bit."

"And that's why I'm pushing forward with this thing. I'm going to nail every one them."

Hawthorn spent the next five minutes telling her what he knew. He told her about Williams and his past,

Gabriella Barcleaves, and the small prescription bottle now tucked inside his coat pocket. When he finished, he asked her to get a vile of Mason's serum from his research pod. They'd need it as proof.

"That's not going to be possible, John."

"What?"

"Mason's pod has been cleaned out."

"What are you talking about?"

"I guess Williams figured he wasn't coming back. One of the other researchers said Williams let a couple of men in there somehow and they took everything. Machines. Vials. Everything."

Hawthorn was crushed. He needed that serum to prove Mason had a legitimate need for the enzyme. Although Mason had sent in his test results months ago, he was still required to provide a final sample to the ICC on the day of the hearing. Without it, he'd be forced to wait six additional months until the next approval hearing.

There was no time to waste. Hawthorn had to move now. He located the blue section in the phone book and dialed the Portland Better Business Bureau. He needed to start small.

Small beads of sweat formed lightly on his brow as the phone rang. In the next five minutes he'd make accusations that could ruin his career. Hawthorn undid the top button on his shirt and took a deep breath. As the phone continued to ring, Hawthorn thumbed past the local government section and into the federal pages. Half way up the third column in black and white, he found an emergency number to the FDA's headquarters in Washington DC.

Hawthorn hung up the phone and dialed the Washington number. He navigated his way through a couple of automated options and got a human on the line.

"FDA. What's the nature of your emergency?"

Hawthorn slouched into the phone, shielding his conversation from another caller four phones down. "I'd like to talk to someone who can receive a very serious issue relating to a major pharmaceutical company."

"Yes, sir. What can I help you with?"

"I am a physician at the CME in Portland, Oregon. I'd like to make a formal plea to remove a company for drug approval consideration."

"Okay, Doctor," the man answered, not really understanding. "What exactly is the nature of your claim?"

"Tomorrow the ICC is holding an approval hearing in San Francisco for several new drugs, one of which is called R2-X. It's been developed by Geniomics based out of Seattle."

"Okay. Please continue."

"I have strong reason to believe that not only have they falsified test results but they may also be tied to several deaths in the Portland area."

"Okay, sir," the man said. There was an uncomfortably long pause. "This is a very serious accusation, doctor."

"John. John Hawthorn," he finished.

"Are any of the alleged parties aware of your knowledge, Dr. Hawthorn?"

"Possibly. Yes. Another physician I work with may know something."

"Okay." Hawthorn could hear the man tapping the keys at his terminal.

"What else can I do?" he asked. "Is there someone local I can go to get some of this down on paper? I really don't know quite what to do here."

"I assure you, sir. This issue will receive top priority. Let's take this one step at a time. How long ago did you find out about this problem?"

"I don't know. Yesterday I suppose."

"Can you give me the name of the substance in question again?"

"R2-X."

"*The* R2-X?" the man asked, surprised.

"Yes, that's it."

There was another long pause on the other end of the line. "Uh, Dr. Hawthorn? Your name is coming up in a box on my screen. There's a message attached to it informing me to call the Office of the Commissioner. Someone else must have reported this as well."

"Good." Hawthorn figured Cindy's friends must have taken the ball and run with it.

"Is there any threat of retaliation, sir?" the man asked. "It's a standard question. No need to worry."

"I really hadn't given it much thought but yes. After what I've seen, I'd say that's a clear possibility."

"And your name is Dr. John Hawthorn. Correct? That's H-A-W-T-H-O-R-N."

"Yes. That's right," answered Hawthorn, anxiously watching a gate representative announcing the boarding plan for his plane. "I apologize, sir, but my plane is about to-"

"All right, Dr. Hawthorn. One moment."

Click.

"Dr. Hawthorn?"

"Yes." Hawthorn watched the mass of people jump into line to board the plane. He'd have to leave very soon.

"I've discussed the matter with one of our chief administrators and, well, we get a lot of calls from people on various things from a headache that never went away to all sorts of stuff I'm sure you don't have time to hear. The point, sir, is that when a person of your stature makes a complaint, we take it very seriously."

"Good. I should hope so."

"Because you may be in some danger by holding this information, I've been instructed to have two agents meet you as soon as possible to escort you to the proper location. I hope that doesn't make you nervous. It's procedure to ensure your safety."

"I understand. I'll be arriving in Portland at 3:45 p.m. from Denver."

"Okay," the man answered, his fingers punching some numbers into his computer. "Everything'll be fine. You're in good hands. Is there anything else I can do for you?"

"I don't think so. I hope some kind of action can be taken before these hearings."

"You'd be surprised how quickly the government can move when we have to."

Hawthorn hung up the phone and sped off to catch his plane.

CHAPTER FORTY

Jordan stepped briskly into the warm sanctity of Hawthorn's apartment to escape the cold Portland air. She removed a long black jacket and laid it neatly across the recliner next to her purse.

"John? You here?" There was no answer. Just like him. What did she expect? That'd he'd actually be there? Whatever. She peered into an empty kitchen.

In the beginning of their relationship, Hawthorn was always on time. He made her feel like she was the only thing he cared for in life. As he got closer to graduating from med school, things changed. Meetings here. Meetings there. Beepers ringing twenty-four hours a day it seemed. Jordan often wondered if Hawthorn would have to one day make a choice between her and his career. It didn't appear he was capable of both.

She walked swiftly around the long, wooden coffee table towards the answering machine. Miracles do happen. Perhaps Hawthorn left a message as to just how late he'd be. She glanced at microwave clock.

"Hello. You have one new message," the machine sounded.

"Finally."

"Uh, John?" said a female voice. Jordan's face turned sour, realizing Hawthorn had failed her yet again. "We may have something. Remember I told you Mason had been clanking vials in the fridge? Well, I didn't have time to take your Slyvy-M measurements yesterday so I took them home and-"

Jordan accidentally hit the 'erase' button, immediately terminating the message. She punched rapidly at a 'save' button hoping to salvage the message but it was too late. Frustrated, Jordan retired to the couch where she contemplated the future. She spun her legs beneath an Afghan and laid her head comfortably on a small throw pillow.

Jordan now realized what it'd be like to have a husband who could be stolen from her at any moment. Not to say that she hadn't given thought to the risks in marrying a doctor. On the contrary, she'd fought through them before and seemed to be getting excellent practice as of late. Then she smiled. He was cute; strong and vulnerable at the same time. And, when he tried, he made her feel on top of the world. She loved his determination and self-reliance. But, then again, the idea of giving your life to someone else was an important decision, one in which Jordan did not want to be wrong.

She grabbed the remote and turned on the television. The first few channels held nothing of interest as she skipped past some meaningless talk shows and news reports. The seconds turned to minutes and the minutes into an hour. Occasionally she'd close her eyes and drift in and out of sleep.

The phone rang loudly from the top of the kitchen counter, startling her. About time.

"John?" There were no sounds coming from the other end. "Hello?"

"Hawthorn," said a man's voice.

"Yes. Hello? You're looking for John?"

"Yes. Is John there?"

"Who is this?"

"Mason."

"Of course. How are you feeling?"

"Tired. I need to go to Vernonia. Is he there?"

"No. As the matter of a fact, he's not," she said, getting herself angry again. "Where are you? I think John's been worried about you."

"Home now. Tired. Had to get away for a bit. I need some help. Are you free?"

"Uh, no. Not really. What for?" Jordan asked, surprised at Mason's directness.

"To retrieve something."

"Heavy?"

"Heavy?" Mason repeated.

"Yeah, heavy. Why else would you need two people?"

"Yes," he answered. "Heavy."

"Is it in storage?"

"I don't- we'll see."

Jordan looked at the clock. She had nothing else to do. "Sure. Why not?" she said, tossing her hand in the air. "How long will we be gone?" She'd leave Hawthorn a note.

"Hard to say. Not long. Depends. Couple of hours."

"Do I need gloves?"

"No you don't. You don't need a thing. Ten minutes."

"Okay. Sounds-"

The line went dead and Jordan placed the portable unit on the table. Mason was so strange. Perhaps he needed someone to talk to not related to the Center. That must be stressful. Hawthorn said he was different. Anyway, if she were there when Hawthorn got back, they'd surely end up in a fight. She needed to get away for a bit. Get out and get some air. Perhaps it'd give her time to cool off and figure out how to tell Hawthorn the big news.

CHAPTER FORTY-ONE

As the travelers before him dispersed into a waiting crowd of friends and family, Hawthorn could see two men in crisp dark suits waiting some distance ahead. Finally. Hawthorn waved.

"Dr. Hawthorn," the first man said, extending his hand. He held out his badge as he introduced himself. "I'm Agent Tasker and this is Agent Madden. We've been instructed to take you to the nearest post."

Tasker, with a square mustache and a face scarred from acne, was the same size as Hawthorn. Madden was as big as a semi. Hawthorn figured him to be at least six foot five and as thick as a bull with arms the size of Hawthorn's legs. Both men concealed side arms beneath straightened suit jackets. He felt protected. Ready to talk.

"This way, sir," said Tasker, motioning towards the main door.

With an officer flanking each side, Hawthorn plowed through criss-crossing travelers. Many of them stared and gossiped as the trio pushed their way onto an escalator that would take them to the car.

As they stepped into the baggage claim area, Hawthorn felt Agent Tasker place his hand just above Hawthorn's elbow. He didn't grasp hard, but he held Hawthorn like a schoolteacher dragging a troublemaker to the principal's office. At the same time, he noticed two members of the airport security team navigating their way through the baggage crowd towards them. Between them marched a heavyset, bald man in a light blue suit. Four or five badges dangled from his neck.

Agent Madden suddenly broke free and headed towards them. Hawthorn paused and, with a nudge on his elbow from Tasker, was urged to continue onward.

"Shouldn't we wait?" Hawthorn asked, slowing a bit.

Tasker nudged him a little harder to quicken the pace. "He'll catch up."

Hawthorn cocked his head sideways to see what the men were doing. The bald man in the blue suit was arguing that airport security officials were to perform escorts inside the building. Apparently, he hadn't been notified and was asking Madden for identification.

"And how was your flight, Dr. Hawthorn?" Tasker asked. They were almost to the door.

"Okay," he answered.

Tasker showed him to an unmarked, blue SUV and after placing Hawthorn's bag in the trunk, unlocked the back door and held it open. He shut the door and circled the car, taking a seat in the driver's position.

Hawthorn peered through the window towards the baggage area. He could see Madden shrugging his shoulders and waving his arms in the air. Tasker, on the other hand, appeared completely unconcerned. He sat nonchalantly in the front seat as if this were the normal course of business.

"Is everything all right?" Hawthorn asked. The rear-view mirror framed perfectly Tasker's dark sunglasses. Hawthorn couldn't tell whether or not he was being watched.

"No need to worry," Tasker replied.

"What's going on in there?" Hawthorn was inching his way further behind the driver's seat.

"Not sure. Airport Security is rarely on top of their game. Shouldn't be long."

Hawthorn straightened his posture and peeked over the edge of the seat, noting the absence of any equipment; no computer or shotgun. Not even a radio. He glanced back towards the building. Madden had finally finished talking and was making his way to the door. As Hawthorn leaned against the seat, he could see that Tasker was sweating.

Hawthorn looked at the lock on his own door. Madden was approaching the vehicle through two sliding glass doors. He opened his door and squeezed his large frame into the passenger's seat. The engine roared as Tasker turned the key.

Suddenly, Hawthorn threw open the back door and exploded from the vehicle. He dodged two taxis and a mini-van and glanced back to see Tasker leaping from the car but unable to cross the thick, slow moving airport traffic. Straight ahead was a large, five-story parking garage.

*   *   *   *   *   *   *   *

"Which way?" Madden asked, pulling his body from inside the car.

Tasker pointed to the gated opening as he watched Hawthorn disappear beneath the first level of the garage. "There. Take the car up the ramp. I'll flush him out."

*   *   *   *   *   *   *   *

Hawthorn flew up the back stairwell to the fourth floor where he quickly sprinted down a car-filled isle. Halfway down the concrete platform, he heard a door slam in the stairwell. He swerved to his left and ducked behind a parked car.

Hawthorn bent his head down and looked beneath a series of car tires. One of them had exited on his floor and was creeping cautiously forward. He rolled over onto his hands and knees and silently backtracked on the front side of the parked cars.

"Come on, Dr. Hawthorn." It was Tasker. "We're here to help."

Clank.

Hawthorn nicked a small metal pipe laying on the ground next to the wall. Both men froze.

*   *   *   *   *   *   *   *

Tasker released the small leather strap holding his firearm in place and stepped carefully between two parked cars. With two hands fastened nervously on the gun's handle, he brushed quietly past the back fender and then past the side doors, bursting around the hood and pointing the barrel to the ground.

There was no one there.

Hawthorn suddenly appeared in a full sprint further up the parking ramp. Tasker raised his gun and fired.

*   *   *   *   *   *   *   *

The silencer chirped and the bullet landed just behind Hawthorn's right leg, lodging itself into the side of nearby car. Hawthorn curled quickly behind the protection of a wide cement column. He reached for his leg as his heart pounded hard beneath his chest.

Hawthorn could hear Tasker approaching. He looked to the ramp one story below and hesitated. Two levels below, Hawthorn could hear the screeching tires of a car speeding up the building's ramp. He was about to get pinched.

Hawthorn scooted along the cement column towards a thick wire that ran along the ramp's edge serving as a stopping point for parking cars. The drop to the next level had to be twelve or thirteen feet. Ten to the car's hood. Tasker was just around the corner. The car was turning onto the ramp beneath him.

*   *   *   *   *   *   *   *

Tasker placed his back to the cement column, his finger tapping lightly against the trigger. His adrenaline was pumping. This is what he loved. Tasker spun hard around the column only to see Hawthorn land loudly on the hood of a parked car one level below. Madden's blue SUV whizzed by and then quickly slammed on its brakes.

Another bullet from Tasker's gun connected with the vehicle's metal hood as Hawthorn spun from the car and jumped to the next level. Madden was already punching the vehicle into reverse, its wheels squealing to position the vehicle back down the ramp. It didn't matter. Hawthorn was hopping entire levels at a time.

Tasker sped his way to the edge of the third level, overlooking the mass of people. Madden jumped from his car with a long, rectangular suitcase and hurriedly assembled a high-powered rifle with a laser guided scope. In a matter of seconds, Hawthorn was between the rifle's cross hairs.

"Right there," whispered Madden. "Good night, doc."

"No," said Tasker.

"I got him." His finger held still on the trigger.

"I said no. Too many people."

"It's gotta be now. He's moving. He'll go inside. It's gotta be now."

Tasker knocked the gun's barrel off target. "We know where he's going." He walked quietly back to the car as Madden watched Hawthorn disappear beneath the safety of the building.

CHAPTER FORTY-TWO

Jordan stood in the kitchen with her hands submerged in a sink full of soap. She glanced at the answering machine for what seemed like the two hundredth time. Hawthorn still hadn't called. The airline told her that the flight had arrived on schedule. "This is ridiculous," she thought. There was absolutely no excuse. And here she was doing his dishes for God's sake. Bullshit.

There was a slight knock at the front door. Jordan slipped the plate gently beneath the suds and dried her hands. She flattened the wrinkles in her shirt and opened the front door. There was no one there. She stepped onto the porch and looked towards the street. Mason was getting back into his car.

"Mason," she called.

He waved his hand for her to join him.

"Be there… in a minute," she said. Jordan returned to the kitchen to turn off the faucet and remove the plug from the bottom of the sink. It' been a long time since she'd been to Vernonia. It was beautiful there. Probably been eight, maybe nine years. The Oregon forest was incredible this time of year. She could hardly wait to take in the fresh open air.

*　　*　　*　　*　　*　　*　　*　　*

Hawthorn pulled urgently alongside the curb across the street from Mason's home. The curtains were pulled shut and the stack of newspapers had grown in number since his last visit. He looked for Mason's car but the garage door was closed.

After inspecting the street for the blue SUV, Hawthorn leapt over a couple of steps and landed on the porch with a loud thud. He rapped hard on the door and rang the doorbell several times. He cupped his hand over his eyes and pressed his face to the bay windows. The blinds had been lowered on this window as well.

"Mason," he called. Hawthorn jumped over a flowerbed at the end of the porch and onto a path that would take him around the backside of the home. He slapped his hand forcefully on another window. "Mason."

Hawthorn felt panicked. There was no telling what he'd find inside. He prayed no one had got to Mason. "Mason," he yelled again.

As Hawthorn searched for another point of entry, he found each window securely locked. Even the back door was tightly fastened by a series of dead bolts. Should he? He looked around. The backyard was fenced in.

Hawthorn stepped back and forcefully kicked at the door near the locked bars. The more he kicked the angrier he became. Finally, the door loosened from its position and, after a barrage of pounding blows, Hawthorn broke through the locks and forced open the door.

He entered a small indoor porch area and glided up two additional steps that led to another door. As he pushed his way through, a horrible aroma sent him reeling backwards, coughing and choking on his own breath. The smell was unbearable. His eyes filled with stinging tears as he hacked and spat to the ground. It felt like his throat was bleeding. Hawthorn grabbed a nearby rag, which he held over his nose and mouth. When he'd finally collected himself, he opened the door and reentered the home.

The kitchen was a mess. Every shelf in the pantry had been emptied and scattered across the ground. Stains of multi-colored liquids scared the walls in uneven blotches. There was an open bin of flour poured everywhere across the ground. Busted canisters and jars had been thrashed and broken about the floor in a complete disaster.

Hawthorn paused. He could hear a faint buzzing sound coming from somewhere in the dimly lit home. With his eyes battling biting tears, Hawthorn stepped carefully over bits and pieces of broken glass. Just ahead on the counter, he could see a clump of spoiled food playing host to a thick army of swarming flies. Their collective buzz sent shivers across his skin.

Hawthorn stopped, his breath quickening.

In the bottom of the sink, he saw what looked like a pail of blood. There was something in there. A solid object was submerged just below the reddish surface. Hawthorn pressed the small towel tighter against his face as his stomach jerked again. A small trail of colored drops lead in an irregular pattern from the sink to the kitchen floor and into the living room.

For a moment, he thought he could see a clump of hair dancing lightly beneath the pool of red. His stomach pulled and Hawthorn suddenly threw up into the bucket of blood. As he moved the towel to vomit, the kitchen's odors quickly found their way to his sense of smell. Hawthorn felt dizzy. He looked at the flies swarming the rotting food and then vomited a second time. One minute later it was over. Just like that. He cleaned his face and pressed the towel again to his mouth.

As he moved cautiously forward into the living room, the small towel dropped to the floor. Mismatched streaks of red ran in jagged strips across the floor and against the far wall. The bookshelves had been cleared of their contents with hundreds of torn pages, papers and books strewn across the floor. Every piece of furniture had been pushed flush against the perimeter of the room.

Hawthorn crept slowly forward. In the middle of the floor was a strange drawing, framed in a crimson square. On the inside were a few crossing lines squiggling from one spot to the next. Hawthorn circled the rectangular shape and squatted close to the floor to examine the dried paste. It looked like blood.

"Mason!" he called again. He could hear a set of wind chimes ringing loudly on the front porch.

Hawthorn's hands were shaking now. He was ready to leave. This was a matter for the police. It was then that Hawthorn noticed that the small trail of drops moved from the base of the drawing, across some texts and journals, and into the darkness of the hallway.

Hawthorn followed the trail from the living room to the edge of the hallway where it disappeared beneath the crack of the bedroom door.

"Mason."

The light was on in the bedroom at the far end of the hall. He sidestepped some broken vases and pictures that had been torn to the ground. Halfway down the hall, he examined a couple of the books and papers that lay destroyed at his feet. Schizophrenia. The next was a paper on visions. There were a couple of books on the interpretation of dreams and an article on memory.

"Mason?"

Hawthorn slowly pushed open the bedroom door. The room was also a catastrophe with more papers and broken trinkets lining the floor. The reddish trail led Hawthorn across the base of the bed, back to the floor, and beneath the closed bathroom door. He could hear the sound of running water.

"Mason. You in there?" Hawthorn walked to the edge of the bathroom door, undecided on what next to do. He could feel himself struggling to breathe in normal rhythm. Again he called Mason's name and then apprehensively nudged open the bathroom door.

A cloud of steam puffed from the small quarters into Hawthorn's face, momentarily blinding his vision. As the cold bedroom air slowly penetrated the tiny room, he could see the faint trail of red scooting across the white tile and beneath a dark blue curtain that protected the tub.

"Mason?" Hawthorn called, inching his way forward. He didn't want to do this. He was making himself move forward one small step at a time. A couple of drops rolled down the side of the bathtub into a small pool of red. Whatever he was about to see hadn't been there long. Hawthorn gathered his courage and pulled the shower curtain to the side.

The severed head of a large black crow floated lazily in a bucket of scalding red water. Its eyes were open and white with decaying skin peeling away from its sockets. Hawthorn covered his mouth and turned off the water.

He flipped open the toilet and fell to his knees. His stomach tightened but for some reason he was unable to vomit. That's when he noticed a small collection of prescription bottles laying on the floor next to a wire-rim wastebasket. He leaned over and picked one up.

They were the pills Mason had developed to facilitate the release of memories. Taking them without a controlling mechanism meant no direction over the release of his subconscious complexes. There was no way to know what to expect.

By Hawthorn's visual count, Mason had exhausted four thirty-count bottles. No wonder it was impossible to connect. *Jesus.* If he thought he was having visions before, Mason just gave his mind a serious boost of adrenaline.

The phone's ring nearly sent Hawthorn to the ground. He shut the bathroom door and scrambled across the bedroom floor, tossing and turning papers and books until he could finally see the phone.

"Hell- Hello. Mason?" Hawthorn's arms trembled as he gripped the portable phone with one of his hands.

"Mason is that you?" The voice was female. "Mason Shane, please. I'm looking for Dr. Mason Shane."

"Dr. Brenner?" Hawthorn inquired.

"John?"

"Yes. Yes. It's me."

"Oh, thank God," she said. "I was so worried that- Is Mason there? I'm very worried about him. I know he hasn't contacted anyone for days."

"I know," said Hawthorn, looking around Mason's room. He put the telephone to his ear and rummaged through some papers on Mason's dresser. "He's in trouble, Dr. Brenner. Big trouble. He's taken some of his own medication. I mean, he's taken a lot."

"The Cyntocin?"

"Yes. His mind must be a tornado right now. I have no idea where he could be." Hawthorn walked back down the hall and into the small study.

"Slow down, John. Take a breath."

"He's in deep trouble. He's in the middle of something at the Center and he can't be thinking clearly right now."

Hawthorn scanned a couple of shelves on the bookcase and then the desk, which appeared unusually clean. A small piece of paper lay centered on its top.

"What is it, John?" Brenner asked.

As Hawthorn reached out to grab the paper, his foot bumped into a small shipping box.

"John?"

"One second." Hawthorn lifted the package to the top part of the desk and examined its exterior. Mason's name and address were there but there was no information on the sender. It'd been mailed a couple of days before from somewhere inside Portland. Hawthorn glanced nervously at the open door. The house was silent. He flipped the package over and saw the hand written words, "Your secret is no more."

Hawthorn poked his fingers through the paper and withdrew the material. Inside was a small stack of newspaper clippings. The first was a story regarding a teenage girl and was dated 1984. Hawthorn almost fainted. She looked exactly like Jordan. Same angling eyebrows. Same jaw line and forehead. Even a slight rounding in the shoulders. The headline noted: "Girl Missing. Police question boyfriend."

"John?" Brenner called. "What is it?"

Hawthorn flipped through a couple of subsequent clippings, which detailed the futile search for the missing girl. He noted the dates. 1984. 1985. After skimming quickly through the first article, he arrived at the boyfriend's name: Mason Shane. Two lines down were some comments from a neurologist who had conducted psychological tests on the young boy. His name was Dr. Allen Williams.

Hawthorn placed the series of articles aside and came across another, older clipping. This one was from 1974 and held two large photographs of a woman and a man. He rifled back to the first clipping. The missing girl. 1984. He flipped back to the woman. 1974. Impossible. They, too, looked strikingly similar in almost every aspect.

Beneath the picture of the woman and man was the photo of a young boy. The headline read: "Boy watches helplessly as mother murders father." The boy was Mason.

"John?"

"Yes... I'm here."

"What are you doing?"

Hawthorn felt like he knew everything and nothing at all. Mason was obviously taking his own drug, which could cause problems by itself, but this. This was an entirely new ball game. This explained why he'd never talked about his parents death; especially his mother. He always said he could never remember her. "She died when I was very young." That's all anyone knew.

Hawthorn didn't know what to do. And here was Brenner on the other end who, for all he knew, could be in the middle of everything.

"Dr. Brenner, I-" Hawthorn paused as he lifted the lone piece of paper from the center of the desk.

"John? John. Are you there, John. What is it?"

Hawthorn walked into the living room. His eyes bounced rapidly between the paper and the floor. What he had once interpreted as some deranged, blood-soaked drawing suddenly took on added significance. Drawn on the small piece of paper was an exact rendition of the painting on the floor. The one exception was a series of small letters and numbers marking each of the squiggling lines on the piece of paper. It was a map. Once Hawthorn could place the abbreviated letters of one road, the others fell quickly into place.

"I'm- I'm sorry," said Hawthorn.

"John, you know I'd do anything to help Mason. Anything. How I can help? Is there something I can do?"

"I'm not sure," Hawthorn answered, dazedly. "I think I know where Mason is."

"I'll go with you."

"No, no. That's not a good idea. He's got to be very... unstable. There's a lot you don't know."

"I'm coming with you, John. West entrance in ten minutes. Everything'll be fine. I can talk to him."

"Please."

"No," Brenner implored. "You be here."

"Fine," answered Hawthorn. "Ten minutes."

CHAPTER FORTY-THREE

Hawthorn arrived at the CME's back entrance with five minutes to spare. He parked his car near the rear loading dock and slipped inside a seldom-used entrance near the base floor. He couldn't chance anything.

"Buddy," Gary said, happily. "Always a pleasure. Always-"

Gary's smile quickly vanished he once saw the look on Hawthorn's face. He nodded to the side door and hit a button to release the lock.

"What's going on?" he whispered. His eyes were bouncing nervously to and from his boss's door in the back of the room.

Hawthorn placed both hands on the desk and leaned in close. "I need more."

"He's here today," Gary answered softly. He looked again to the door.

Hawthorn lowered his head. A group of people were moving through the adjacent hall just outside Gary's small window. "I need to see Mason's file."

"John, I can't just-" Gary's boss walked out of his office and into the room, scratching the top part of his head and then covering his yawning mouth. He grabbed a stack of papers and returned to his office. "I can't. Purchasing info, maybe, but I can't get personal records. I don't have clearance. Only Williams and Beltman can get in."

"What? A password?"

"Yes."

"Let's give it a shot. Dial it up."

Gary looked to his boss's door and then reluctantly booted up the program. Two seconds later the screen prompted him for a password. He shrugged his shoulders. "Two minutes, John. That's it."

Hawthorn closed his eyes, thinking. "Try Williams' middle name. If that doesn't work, let's try his birthday."

Gary's fingers danced across the keys. Access denied. "This is ridiculous. The odds are enormous."

"How about Geniomics?" Hawthorn spelled it out letter by letter. That didn't work either. "Try his social security number. It's on that sheet right there."

Gary looked at a nearby document and entered the numbers. No response. "It's probably something close to him. You know, a secret. Maybe his mother's or his father's birthday."

"Try Mullin. Or Samantha."

Gary typed in the word Mullin. This, too, didn't work. "Hawthorn, I'm telling you. It could be anything."

"Try Barcleaves."

Gary gave him a frustrated look and then typed in the letters. Bingo.

"Okay – pull up Mason's file."

Gary glanced nervously to his boss's door. "Hawthorn, come on, man. I could get busted."

"Do it Gary. Let's go."

Gary searched the personnel files for Mason's name and then brought up his file on the screen. Hawthorn's eyes moved quickly across the bits of information. The amount of available data was incredible. There was everything from psychological profiles to fitness tests. In other sections there was information ranging from historical physiological information to notes on each person's research.

"Here," said Hawthorn, his finger pointing to the section containing psychological treatment and therapy.

Gary tapped the button and up popped a dated list of various tests and therapy in which Mason had been involved. As promised, he'd undergone testing in neurology a couple of days before. Their tests showed traces of Cyntocin in his bloodstream. Williams was obviously aware that Mason was consuming his own medication.

"Scroll down," Hawthorn commanded, his finger touching the list of dates.

Gary scrolled the screen from top to bottom as Hawthorn's eyes rolled past each date. Hawthorn's brow tensed as the sheer number of dates indicated that Mason had been receiving an extensive volume of therapy for the past several years. At the very end was what he assumed to be the very first date of Mason's treatment.

Hawthorn anxiously rubbed his forehead. Whereas each of the other entries contained a subject line to give the reader an idea of the therapy involved, this one was blank. Its date was September 23, 1984, several years before the next entry. With Hawthorn's persuasion, Gary tapped the link and brought up a private report written by Dr. Williams himself.

Hawthorn sped over the details of Williams' narration, which recounted his own examination of a 17-year old Mason Shane. Apparently Williams, a practicing neurologist and psychologist at the time, was asked to profile Mason after a young girl was reported missing. By Hawthorn's own perception, Williams had commissioned several private and illegal psychological tests that included narcotic-induced hypnotism and guided imagery, none of which would have been admissible in court.

Evidently, Mason showed no recollection of his whereabouts for nearly a week's time. He complained of nausea, dizziness, and extensive blackouts. What Williams did with the results was anyone's guess but his report showed Mason to suffer from dissociative identity disorder combined with severe posttraumatic stress and spontaneous hypermnesia, a condition that could elevate historical trauma in a moment's notice.

Hawthorn went on to read that during one of the hypnosis sessions, another physician used guided imagery and deep hypnosis to take Mason back in time. Apparently, Mason elevated a spontaneous abreaction, suddenly exploding emotionally to an event with his mother. The physicians were able to isolate his mother's presence in triggering suppressive anger. Evidently, Mason was reliving the trauma as if it were happening in the present.

Hawthorn tightened the muscles in his jaw and clenched his teeth. No wonder Williams buried the fact that Mason had taken his own drug. Without a managing device, he knew exactly what kind of problems would find their way to the surface.

"Yikes," said Gary, reading a few of the lines at the top of the screen. "Did you know about this?"

Hawthorn's veins turned to ice. Cindy was to meet Xiao that afternoon. He picked up the phone and called the lab. There was no answer. He called her at home.

"Hello?" Her voice sounded immediately urgent.

"Cindy, listen to me."

"Hawthorn, I left something for you at-" There was some rustling noise in the background. Then the line went dead.

*   *   *   *   *   *   *   *

Hawthorn burst into the living room of his apartment and found it completely trashed. The cushions on the furniture had been torn to pieces and every shelf emptied to the ground. Even the drawers in a small desk were emptied and tossed about the room. The kitchen was worse. The refrigerator door was open with all of its contents strewn across the tile. Smashed eggs. Broken glasses and plates. Pools of milk and juice.

"Jordan?!"

Hawthorn raced to the back of the apartment, passing the coffee table in the living room where his research log books were arranged haphazardly across the flat surface.

"Jordan!" he yelled, running to the bedroom. "Jordan!"

The study was empty as was the bedroom and each closet. Hawthorn checked the bathroom and then moved to a second bathroom located in the main hall. It, too, was empty, but as Hawthorn withdrew himself to run back to his car, he noticed something sitting behind a box of Kleenex. It was a small tube, open at one end and closed at the other. Half was red and half of it blue. Hawthorn knew exactly what it meant.

He scrambled through some trash to locate the box and then raced his finger down its side to interpret the results. Jordan was pregnant. Hawthorn was going to be a father. His stomach sank with fear as he thought of what they might have done with her. Hawthorn slammed his fist against the cabinet. He felt sick that he hadn't warned her.

Perhaps she'd been gone. Yes. She'd have left a note. Jordan always left a note. As he frantically unearthed a stack of papers on his kitchen counter, Hawthorn noticed the small light blinking rapidly on his answering machine.

"John? Going with Mason to Vernonia. Be back by six."

*　　*　　*　　*　　*　　*　　*　　*

Mason's car traveled quickly down the small two-lane highway to Vernonia. The scenery was fabulous with tall evergreens lining the road and lush undergrowth dotting the base of each towering pine.

Although Jordan and Mason had spoken while driving through the outskirts of Portland, no words had been exchanged for nearly fifteen minutes. Something else was on his mind. His eyes had been scanning the right side of the road for the past ten minutes.

"Have you ever wondered who you really are?" Mason asked. He glanced out through the driver's window and then stared at the road ahead. He hadn't looked at her the entire trip.

"My mom always said I was a trouble maker. Then again, I'm sure she'd argue that's who I really am," Jordan answered, trying to lighten the conversation. Mason didn't flinch. "Why?"

"Is it really possible to know everything about yourself? Don't you wonder if we keep secrets even from ourselves?"

"Sure," she said, glancing through her own window at the passing roadside. "Maybe there are some things we don't want to know. Or shouldn't. The truth hurts, right?"

Another five minutes of silence passed. Jordan tried everything to jump-start the conversation, but Mason simply wouldn't budge. She asked about his project and his hobbies and each time she received no acknowledgment of her question. The deadening silence was making her more and more uncomfortable.

"Have you ever done something completely out of character?" Mason asked. Again, the question seemed to come out of nowhere. "You can't explain it but it's as if, for a moment, you were a completely different person."

A weathered, green road sign indicated there were still twenty miles to go. Jordan couldn't wait to get out of the car. Suddenly, Mason slammed on the brakes and swerved the vehicle onto a small dirt road that led into the thick Oregon forest.

"What are you doing?" she asked, now gripping the door handle of his car.

*   *   *   *   *   *   *   *

"Where could they be?" Brenner asked. They were ten miles outside of Portland and Hawthorn had his car pushing its limits for speed. Next to him, resting on the console was Mason's map. He glanced to its numbers and crossing lines to ensure the proper direction.

"I know how you're feeling, John," Brenner said. "I feel the same. Mason's life has been difficult to say the least. Do you know anything about his past?"

Hawthorn's mind drifted to the articles. He had his own suspicions. "I know of his grandfather and that he had trouble with his parents."

Hawthorn swerved to the left to pass a slower moving car. He didn't want to admit what he knew regarding Mason's childhood or parents just yet.

"His mother was a sick woman. Very sick. She suffered not only from alcoholism but dissociative identity disorder. Never once received treatment for it."

"That's hereditary."

"Yes," she answered. "She was beaten severely by her own parents when she was young. Mason's mother committed suicide in the Oregon state mental institution when he was still very young."

Hawthorn focused on the road ahead and he pushed the accelerator to the floor.

"It was awful," she continued. "Apparently she killed his father one afternoon in a manic rampage. They had a fight. Child comes home. Father slips. She sticks him with a knife. Mason survived by hiding under a table, but saw the entire thing."

"And then he goes to live with his grandfather."

"Right. When I learned of his story and how he was able to overcome this tragedy to become a brilliant student, I used all of my influence to get him to attend Stanford. Dr. Williams was quite impressed with his brilliance."

For the next fifteen or twenty miles, Hawthorn explained everything to her. She was unaware of Mason's involvement with the missing girl some fifteen years before or his history with Williams shortly thereafter. She was not surprised. People with his condition, she explained, could enter an emotional state and then regain consciousness as if nothing ever happened.

Of course, this meant that each time he met someone with similar characteristics to his mother, Mason could potentially relive its nightmarish past. There was no way to know what could touch it off. The missing girl obviously had never been found. Hawthorn thought of Jordan and then pressed the gas pedal hard to the floor.

*　　*　　*　　*　　*　　*　　*　　*

Mason's car bounced and rocked along a primitive dirt road, slicing its way higher and higher into the pine-covered Oregon mountains. The Bronco's wheels rode high on the outside edges of deeply cut grooves where mud had been parted by another vehicle and then dried by the sun.

Jordan questioned Mason's choice of direction for a few minutes and then realized he wasn't going to talk. He remained silent, his eyes picking apart the forest's edge. She considered opening the door and jumping out. What then? The car was moving too quickly. She quietly reached into a handbag and saw that her cell phone had no service. Each minute in that Bronco took her further and further away from civilization. She had to do something.

"Mason? I-I really think we should turn around. This road is going nowhere. Maybe this is the wrong way." Mason pinched his forehead with his hand as if he were experiencing some pain. What could he be looking for? There was nothing out here.

By Jordan's estimate, they were ten miles into the forest. From the clock on Mason's dash, they'd turned off of the highway at 5:06 and it was now 5:34.

Fifty yards ahead, Jordan could see the ground beneath the road break upwards forming a natural speed bump. He'd have to slow down. This was her chance. She scanned the door handle and lock to plan her escape. "I'd really like for you to stop the vehicle, Mason. You're scaring me," she pleaded.

The bump was just ahead. Mason pressed down on the gas pedal causing the vehicle to accelerate forward. She gripped the underside of her seat. He wasn't slowing down.

"Here," shouted Mason. He slammed on the brakes and the car slid to a stop, the tires inches from the hump. Mason took the keys and exited the vehicle. He pushed the driver's seat forward and grabbed a military shovel, which he extended to its full length. Mason slammed the door and headed towards the trees.

Jordan locked her door and nervously followed his image around the back of the car in her side view mirror. He wasn't waiting for her. She cracked the window. "Where are you going?" she called.

Mason mumbled something unintelligible as he continued towards the forest's edge. His right hand gripped the shovel tightly as he plowed his way between a thick patch of thorns and a tree's extending branches.

"What are you doing?" she yelled.

Mason stopped and tipped the shovel's blade towards her. "I know who you are. I know exactly who you are."

As Mason disappeared into the Oregon timberland, Jordan sat alone in the vehicle's cockpit fearfully inspecting the darkening landscape. She scrambled through her purse and withdrew her cell phone. Still no service. She couldn't tell whether it was more frightening to be alone in the vehicle or to be out there with Mason. It'd be pitch black by the time she could travel a quarter of the way back to the highway. She had to stay with him. At this point it was more important to know exactly where he was. After a minute or so, she broke from the car and headed into the forest.

Despite having closed the gap considerably between her and Mason, Jordan now moved delicately forward. Her feet were on fire and ached from her sandal's leather straps, which carved their position into her skin. She stopped and gazed into the forest, barely able to make out the back of Mason's shirt bobbing in and out of the distant trees. In every direction the earth was spotted with small patches of light and the once blue sky had now turned to the dark underside of towering branches crossing high overhead.

"Mason," Jordan yelled. He was now completely out of sight. "Mason!"

Her ankle wobbled sideways as one of the straps pulled free from a buckle on her sandal. *Damn it.* These were her favorite pair of shoes. A gift from her father from Spain. She yanked off the buckle and threw it angrily towards a couple of trees. Jordan tucked the dangling strap beneath another crossing section of her sandal and cursed. She looked at the display of her cell phone. Nothing.

Jordan had no idea which way to go. The forest looked the same in every direction. She listened carefully. Occasionally a strong gust of air would blow through the branches but, for the most part, there were no audible clues. She wiped the sweat from her brow. Perhaps she should find the road and try to make it home. She just wanted to leave.

For the next hundred yards, it seemed, the land rose and fell like a soft rolling blanket. She'd travel slowly up one hill only to move gradually down the next. After a brief period of flat terrain, Jordan descended a small embankment. The ground was damp and sank slightly beneath each step as she navigated carefully around several ferns and fallen logs. At the bottom of the ravine she paused. Somewhere in the distance she could hear the faint sounds of a metal blade pounding the earth.

Mason.

A faint path appeared to lead beneath a thick grouping of trees, which rose from the ground like a man-made dam. The closer she approached, the more she could see that the path did not end, rather it continued through a small hole in a curtain of branches.

"Mason?" she called again. The digging sounds continued. She squatted down and looked through the narrow opening.

The dirt path beneath her feet, a deer path most likely, led into a natural tunnel of trees whose dense connecting branches overhead formed a perfect cathedral of arches. At the other end, Jordan could see a beautiful quilt of grass illuminated brightly by the direct rays of the sun. She stood and looked the other way, back down the ravine. Then she glanced to the sky. Jordan slipped through the opening and into the shaded tunnel of trees.

At the end of the tunnel Jordan stopped and hid herself quietly behind one of the bordering trees. Mason was swinging the shovel wildly into the forest soil as he grunted and struggled for each breath. Next to him were four evenly spaced stones that seemed to mark the center of the sunlit clearing.

"Claire, Claire, Claire," he yelled. Mason's shirt was drenched with sweat and his pants covered in blotches of dirt. Between words he would slam the shovel deeper and deeper into the ground.

Suddenly, Mason stopped. He looked up at the tips of the towering pines as if he were listening to someone speak. His head spun in each direction. He mumbled something to the sky. Suddenly enraged, he pounded the metal blade harder into the earth.

"Leave me alone," he snarled. "Get out of here, boy."

The shovel's blade suddenly clanked loudly against something solid. He tossed the blade aside and, with his bare hands, scratched frantically at the soft earth inside the pit. "Who am I?" he yelled. "Do you know? Will anyone know?"

Jordan had seen enough. Mason was boxed in a frenzy. Fearing for her life, she moved quickly down the path away from the clearing. From there she would find the road and follow it back to the main highway. It didn't matter how long it took.

"I put you there," she heard Mason yell. "Get-out-of-my-life!"

*   *   *   *   *   *   *   *

Mason suddenly hooked his fingers on a red-checkered piece of cloth, pulling it free from the earth. He jerked back in terror as the cloth tore apart, exposing a smaller skeletal hand.

He let out a terrible scream.

The faint sound of a broken branch suddenly caught his attention. He glanced down the pathway. A woman was nearing the end.

"Claire!" he screamed wildly. Mason picked up the shovel and ran angrily down the darkened corridor, swinging violently at the branches that lined his way.

CHAPTER FORTY-FOUR

Crazy what people will do in a panic. For many, their physical being freezes; labored breathing, dizziness, and headaches tear at their senses like a biting arctic winter. For others it is a call to arms; adrenaline flows forcefully through every pore in the body, causing the mind to heighten its awareness and the physique to push forth with great agility and strength. For John Hawthorn it was desperation. There were few clues left on Mason's map whose crude blueprint had guided Hawthorn successfully along two connecting highways, three logging roads, and finally onto a rocky forest service route seamlessly absorbed by the primitive, old-growth forest.

Ten miles into Oregon timberland, Hawthorn's small car came to a skidding halt. Mason's Bronco was parked twenty yards ahead. Hawthorn and Brenner exited the vehicle and met around back to take one final look at the map.

"What do you think?" Brenner asked, gazing across the army of trees. She had fear in her eyes, now exposed in open air.

Hawthorn flipped the map around in his hands. There was no more information to be had. This was it. "I have no idea. Let me see your watch."

Brenner pulled up her sleeve, exposing the timepiece. Hawthorn then rolled up his own sleeve and placed his watch next to hers. "Okay. Here's what has to happen."

Brenner was staring tensely at the edge of the forest.

"Doctor," he said again. Brenner slowly zeroed in. "Are you okay?"

She nodded.

"Okay." He pointed across the top of the car. "You take that way. Walk for ten minutes then turn to your right and walk for another ten. Ninety degree turns."

"Make a square."

"Right. Just keep yelling for them. They couldn't have gone far. They have to hear us."

"Okay."

"I'm going that way," he said, pointing in the opposite direction. "I'm sure we'll find them. Okay? Forty minutes."

*   *   *   *   *   *   *   *

Brenner paused at the edge of the forest to see Hawthorn running full speed beneath the trees. Occasionally he would hop to his right and left as he bobbed his way in and out of the forest's obstacles. When he was finally out of sight, she turned around and began her own reluctant quest for the missing couple.

*   *   *   *   *   *   *   *

Hawthorn was determined to make the most of his forty minutes. The landscape to his side blurred as it went speeding past. He would travel at top speed until a cramp in his lungs forced him to rest. At each break he would stop and call out their names.

"Jordan!"

With the first leg of his sprint complete, Hawthorn rested momentarily with his hands on top of his knees. He was surprised at his lack of stamina. He used to be able to run that distance with no problem. Hawthorn stretched upright and took in a deep breath. The elevation was killing him. Even worse, it appeared as if the landscape ahead sloped up-

Hawthorn noticed a slight glimmer twenty feet to his side. *A buckle.* He lifted it from the ground and gave it a closer look. He'd seen it before. Jordan's shoes. Hawthorn let out a desperate laugh. Another gift from her father. She couldn't stop talking about them.

The joy, however, quickly returned to fear. He had no idea which direction they'd gone. Hawthorn tried to imagine from where the strap could have been thrown. He had to take a chance. He was running out of time.

A few more minutes of sprinting and Hawthorn slowed to regain his breath. He stood at the top of a small ditch filled densely with moss-coated trees and their criss-crossing branches.

"Jordan!" His voice echoed through the forest. "Mason!"

Hawthorn looked down the slope at the wall of trees. Hawthorn realized he'd lose his direction and timing if he tried to go around them. He had to maintain direction to complete the square. He'd go through the trees and double his speed on the other side.

Skipping quickly down the hill and then moving slowly through the first part of the dense foliage, Hawthorn took extra time to move the heavy branches from his way. Each step was carefully placed over the fallen logs and uneven ground. Within moments, Hawthorn found himself standing at the midpoint of what appeared to be a tunnel beneath the trees. At one end of the small corridor was an outlet leading to the rest of the ravine. The other end opened to sunlit carpet of swaying green grass. He could see footprints dotting the soft dirt in both directions. Hawthorn glanced down the ravine and then sprinted towards the circle of light.

As he broke through the darkness of trees, Hawthorn's heart jumped. Protruding from the freshly dug pit was a skeletal hand that rested comfortably on the edge of the grave. He knew instantly who it was.

"Mason!" he shouted.

Hawthorn inspected the circumference of trees eventually coming full circle to the tunnel. From this vantage point he could see a jagged pattern of broken branches leading down the thin corridor. Fear and anger stung him with the thought of what may lie ahead.

The trail of broken branches led Hawthorn up one side of the trench and back into the forest. Every twenty or thirty yards he could see pockets of smashed tree limbs that helped guide him along. Hawthorn skipped lightly across the earth, speeding precariously forward in search of his fiancée. With each guiding clue came the hope that Jordan was alive and the fear that Mason was not far behind.

Hawthorn looked briefly ahead, unable to locate the next lead. His pace quickly diminished as he looked in every direction for the next sign.

Thirty yards away, beyond the end of a fallen log, extended a tress of soiled blonde hair. Hawthorn's stomach surged and his breath became short and fatigued. She wasn't moving. His knees wobbled as he stepped forward with great apprehension.

The short distance felt like a lifetime of movement. Time and space slowed as Hawthorn floated helplessly towards the body. He feared the pain Mason had inflicted upon her. A million lost moments raced through his head as he fell to his knees on the opposite side of the log. He couldn't bring himself to look at her. He couldn't bear to see her face.

Hawthorn wiped the tears from his eyes and gazed once more at the golden hair in the palm of his hand. He wanted to cement her picture in his mind so that he would never remember this moment.

Naaaajon.

At first he thought the sound to be the forest wind but soon recognized the chime of a human voice. Jordan.

Hawthorn peered over the log. It was Brenner. She'd taken a strong blow to the side of her head. He removed his jacket and placed it neatly across the top of the log so that someone would easily find her body. Hawthorn then locked on to the distant voice and rushed frantically into the darkening trees.

After battling the turbulent, mountainous landscape, Hawthorn arrived at the parked cars. His body jerked backwards at the edge of the trees. The number of cars parked in the crude forest clearing had grown to three. Located next to Mason's vehicle was another car. A blue SUV.

Aaaatthonnn.

Hawthorn whipped around, listening intently for the sound of Jordan's voice. He tilted his head to get a better read with the wind. They were near, perhaps on the other side of a nearby ridge. Hawthorn crept quietly along the edge of the forest and then sprinted frantically off in a new direction.

CHAPTER FORTY-FIVE

For the past several minutes, Jordan had desperately fought her way up and down the treacherous lengths of the rolling land. Each time she was forced to climb, the muscles in her bony legs would quiver and shake from fatigue. And each time, just as she was about to collapse, the terrain would flatten and she would regain her will to survive.

Jordan paused to see Mason climbing the side of a ditch twenty seconds behind. He was rapidly closing the gap between them. Just as Jordan had pushed her frame to its physical limits, so had Mason, raging forward and swinging wildly at anything in his path.

Jordan pumped her arms harder and concentrated on revolving her legs faster and faster. There was a small passageway cutting through the wall of a large rock formation just ahead. She glanced behind and then bounced over a fallen tree that angled towards the ground. He was now twenty, maybe thirty, yards behind.

Jordan burst through the narrow opening and then traveled fleetly down a steep slope towards a creek. Her footsteps plowed through the ice-cold stream and, once safely across, followed along the banks of the flowing brook. She glanced across the stream. Mason was taking a higher route along a ten-foot ledge on the other side of the creek. As he danced from rock to rock, she could see his eyes bouncing between the narrow path on which he moved and herself, struggling through the thick brush to survive. He was looking for a way down.

Jordan lowered her head and threw out her arms in a makeshift shield as branches crashed all around her. She could barely feel her legs. The freezing water had numbed them from the tips of her toes all the way to her knees.

Jordan glanced at the ledge again and paused. Mason was gone. She'd lost him through the trees. Where was he? It was nearly impossible to discern one object from the next. The cold and pain was affecting her ability to focus.

That's when she saw him. Mason was crossing the creek just ahead. He held the shovel high above his head as he plowed through the water towards her. Jordan immediately left the creek's edge and scrambled up the side of a steep hill. For each foot she climbed, the soft earth took six inches. Eventually, she reached the top, just seconds ahead of Mason.

Jordan bounced to one side to avoid an oncoming tree. She could hear his labored breathing between the smashing swings of his shovel as he drew closer.

Suddenly, the smashing ceased. Jordan curved to her right, still traveling at top speed. The ground appeared to even from here to the next incline, something she needed desperately as she wheezed and coughed.

Out of the corner of her eye, Jordan noticed something slanting quickly towards her. He was trying to cut her off. In an instant, Jordan lowered herself and accelerated forward.

She could feel her balance shifting as his nails dug hard into the back of her neck and then ripped across the sleeve of her shirt. Jordan spun sideways and circled to the opposite side of a nearby tree. Mason had already regained his balance. For the next ten seconds they mimicked each other's moves. Each time Mason bobbed right, Jordan would jerk quickly to her right to keep the tree between them.

"Mason, stop it," she cried. Her long blonde hair was straightened with sweat and her arms covered in bruises and small cuts. "Why are you doing this?"

"Get out," Mason snarled. He raised the shovel and swung hard at her hands. Jordan jerked back and surveyed the landscape, ready to make another escape. Mason yanked the shovel from the tree's side.

"Please," she begged.

Mason swung again, this time dislodging the bark just above Jordan's fingers. She shuffled frantically around the tree's base as he cocked back and swung a third time. Again, Jordan pulled back and the blade stuck deep into the trunk of the tree. Using its handle as a slingshot, Mason lunged desperately towards her, again grabbing the material on her shoulder. She yelled at the top of her lungs and punched his arm away. Mason retreated and grabbed hold of the shovel's handle. He pulled with all of his might as Jordan whirled about and ran for her life.

As she weaved through ferns, boulders and a maze of trees, Jordan glanced at her feet, somehow scrambling knowingly across the obstacle-laden earth. Thorns and branches had long ago torn through the skin on her legs and she now found her shins bleeding and her thighs dull with pain.

Jordan climbed a small incline into what looked like a break in the forest. A huge clearing. She desperately needed the flat terrain. Not only were her legs numb and tattered with criss-crossed lacerations, but her lungs felt scorched by each gasping breath she'd taken to survive. She needed help. Her body was winding down. At the top of the hill, she broke past some thick brush and slid to a halt.

Just ahead the mountainous landscape abruptly dropped, displaying a vast wooded valley below. At the bottom of the purple sky was another set of mountains perhaps some twenty miles away with thin bands of clouds hovering just above the tree line in white, horizontal sheets.

Jordan wavered. She was cornered. Her heart quickened. She couldn't tell from where she had entered. Mason should have been there by now. He was waiting. Watching. Jordan moved cautiously to the edge of the cliff and peered carefully over its side. Immediately, she pulled back. The drop was a hundred feet or more.

Jordan gasped and slowly backpedaled and then saw Mason standing silently at the edge of the trees. The long battle with the Oregon woods had blackened his garments with dark shades of soil and plant and his shirt, once a white sheet of cloth, was now torn and stained with fresh blotches of earth and blood.

Jordan could see the shovel's tip covered in red. There were fragments of blonde hair clumped together on the edge of the blade. Someone had come for her. Someone had come for her and someone had died. Jordan suddenly felt helpless. There was nowhere to go. It was over.

With shovel sitting evenly between two bloodied hands, Mason stalked gradually forward. His blackened eyes locked on hers.

Jordan retreated further to the cliff's edge. She was sobbing now. "Mason, please. I don't want to die," she begged.

Mason gritted his teeth and breathed heavily through his mouth like an angry lion preparing an attack. "Damn you, Claire," Mason snapped. "Pain. And Hate. And Death."

Jordan arched over her stomach as Mason swung the shovel towards her mid section. She glanced behind. The edge of the cliff was four feet away.

"I haven't done anything, Mason. Who are you talking to?" she sobbed. "I'm Jordan. It's me." At the edge of the cliff, she sank to the ground and curled into a small ball around her ankles for protection.

Mason loomed over her, the shovel extending from his right hand. He nudged the back of her head with the tip of the shovel. "Get up."

Jordan buried her head deep into her arms, crying uncontrollably. "Please. I haven't done-"

"I said, get up, Claire!" Mason's voice boomed through the forest. His face was tensed with newfound anger.

Jordan tried to stand but her muscles would barely hold her up. Pieces of rock and dirt tumbled over the edge of the cliff as she cringed ever closer to the land's end.

"Back to hell," he said abruptly. Mason raised the shovel high overhead to deliver the final blow. "Back to hell, you drunk-"

*   *   *   *   *   *   *   *

"Mason!" Hawthorn stood at the edge of the trees, inching his way forward.

Mason paused, apparently confused, his mind lost between a world of insanity and illusion and the real people in his life. As he struggled to make the connection, Mason lowered the shovel from above his head.

Hawthorn moved delicately forward. "I'm here now, Mason. You don't have to do this. Please put it down." He was ten feet away and could see Mason's eyebrows crest as if he were showing signs of recognition. "Come on, Mason. Let's go home."

"Home," Mason growled. A look of rage swept suddenly across his face. He raised the shovel angrily overhead, spinning towards Jordan.

"No!" Hawthorn yelled, rushing towards the edge of the cliff. Hawthorn slammed Mason hard to the ground as Jordan scrambled quickly beneath the safety of the trees.

Mason twisted his body from beneath Hawthorn's frame, flipping him easily onto his back. He pinned one of Hawthorn's arms to the ground as his hand scrambled across the nearby earth for a baseball-size rock.

Hawthorn stretched out his arms to block the downward trajectory of Mason's raging blow. He could feel a couple of ribs snap and pop in different directions.

Mason swung the rock again causing Hawthorn to wheeze loudly as his breathing was abruptly interrupted a second time.

"Mason," Jordan called from the forest's edge. She tried to stand, but her legs would not cooperate.

Hawthorn cocked back with a free arm and punched hard at Mason's jaw, rocking him slightly off balance. He struggled to regain his position, but Mason was still in control. Mason drew back his own arm and landed a blow flush against the side of Hawthorn's face, tearing open the flesh around his lips.

The more they battled, the more blood that seemed to find its way into Hawthorn's eyes. Soon enough, he could only make out the darkened shapes of Mason's oncoming fist as they slammed into the sides of his face and body. Mason landed another punch. Then another. Hawthorn was losing the battle. And another. He could barely make out the hollowing sounds of Jordan's voice as she cried helplessly from the edge of the trees.

Mason freed himself as Hawthorn now laid defenselessly battered near the cliff's edge. Mason stumbled backwards a few steps and regained his shovel.

"No," cried Jordan.

Mason held the weapon loosely overhead, his face filled with rage.

"Boone," Hawthorn mumbled, his words followed by coughs of blood that caused him to wheeze in pain. This was his last chance. He had to play Mason's game.

Mason again appeared confused. "What?" He dropped the shovel to his side and kneeled beside Hawthorn's beaten frame.

"Shepard Boone."

"Boone?" Mason asked, his attention now locked on Hawthorn's swollen, bloodshot eyes. "Boone."

Hawthorn creased at the waist as a glob of bloodied drool seeped from his mouth.

Mason rocked back on his heels as if he'd reached a pinnacle of understanding. His face lightened as he stood and moved back to the edge of the cliff, pondering this new information. "Boone."

Hawthorn rolled painfully onto his side, his ribs shifting in abnormal directions. He climbed slowly to his elbows and could feel the water in his swollen eyelids rotate with gravity's pull. He looked to Jordan who stared vacantly back at him in a state of shock.

As Mason paced along the cliff's edge, Hawthorn could see a small dot of red light suddenly appear on the back of Mason's shirt. It jiggled back and forth and then followed his spine to the middle of his head. It was coming from the edge of the trees.

"Mason," Hawthorn coughed out in pain.

The gun's exploding bullet chirped loudly through the valley as Mason disappeared over the edge of the cliff. Hawthorn clung to the ground, scrambling to find cover. Jordan broke from the edge of the trees, somehow finding the energy to throw herself across him.

Far in the distance, Hawthorn could see angling beams of white light as a search and rescue team moved quickly their way. As Jordan sobbed and clutched at his tired physique, Hawthorn could see the small red dot traveling up the back of Jordan's leg.

"No!" Hawthorn yelled, pulling her tightly against him. The red circle of light was moving towards the middle of her back. Jordan clutched him harder.

Suddenly, the beam of light disappeared and was followed by some debate from the edge of the trees. As fast as it had gone, the powerful red light blinded Hawthorn in one eye. He clutched hard at Jordan's arms. He could see his father and mother. His wife and child. Hawthorn squeezed his eyes and waited. Again the light disappeared and Hawthorn could hear two men fleeing along the forest's edge.

Thirty seconds later, Hawthorn was illuminated by a distant beam of light. The oncoming rescue team split quickly in two, as half of them pursued the fugitives while the others found their way to the battered couple.

"I'm sorry," Hawthorn said. "I'm so sorry." As Jordan wept against his shoulder, Hawthorn could see a small piece of paper resting on the ground nearby. It had fallen from Mason's pocket during the struggle. He stretched painfully forward and gathered it in his hand.

Hawthorn unfolded the paper. It was a note written in a youthful script and was dated 1984. This was the note Mason had read to him in the cemetery. "To whomever finds this note. I make no excuses for what I've done. Fate has not been kind to me. I was led to the path I have taken. Funny how little choice we have over the direction of our lives. I have seen many pass before me and have spoken in many voices. And always I have tried to heal the wound within me. I write these words, hoping, perhaps futilely, that I will see them again when I return. When I am healed. Bearcloud is near."

Jordan kissed him on the side of the head as he looked coldly into the half-circle of trees.

"It was the only way he could explain what he had done to that girl. It was the only way he could explain what his mother had done to his father."

In a matter of minutes, the rescue team had arranged for their transportation to safety. Jordan was taken by ambulance to the local hospital where she was treated for exhaustion and minor contusions. Hawthorn, given time to rest and recover, refused immediate care. Instead, he led the team to Brenner's body. He thanked them for their work and graciously accepted a ride back to the hospital where he would gather some of his own research. The pain no longer mattered. He had to piece something together for the ICC hearing the next day. Hawthorn was determined to run both Geniomics and Williams into the ground.

*   *   *   *   *   *   *   *

Flanked by two patrolmen, Hawthorn limped painfully across the CME atrium towards the information booth. Mabel nervously withdrew a pencil from her silver hair and looked him over uneasily.

"Hawthorn, my goodness, what's happened to you?" she asked, grabbing for the phone. "Let me call someone."

Hawthorn placed his finger on the button. "Is Williams in?"

"I-I don't know. I suppose I can check his on line calendar." She tapped a couple of buttons on her computer and brought up William's schedule. "No, he's in San Francisco tonight and tomorrow. Is there something I can help you with?"

"I need to get to my research. Williams changed my access. I have no other way of getting to it."

Mabel hesitated, and then looking him over once again, handed him her badge. She had clearance to deliver mail to the fourth floor. Hawthorn squeezed her hand and mouthed the words 'thank you'.

Everything inside Mason's pod was gone. There were no machines, no cabinets, and no refrigeration devices. Hawthorn traveled into the lab towards the back of the fourth floor. Several vials and glass bowls had been shattered. Books and journals had been emptied from the library with their pages torn from the binders. Even the padlock on his own refrigeration unit was missing, as were the vials and other containers that held Hawthorn's Slyvy-M research. He searched the counters for a copy of his data log. If nothing else, he could use its contents to show other tests on the enzyme. Hawthorn thrashed through a pile of paper and then realized that it, too, had disappeared.

He shouted, throwing some papers across the room. The two officers said nothing and waited quietly behind.

Hawthorn slumped into a nearby stool. He felt devastated. There was nowhere to go. He picked up a broken vial and read the label. It was from the Slyvy-M project. He could hear a door slam closed in the distance. Beltman was approaching with his own entourage of security personnel.

"We can file a report if you'd like, Dr. Hawthorn," one of the nearby officers said. "We'll be right outside."

"Thanks," Hawthorn replied. He looked at the ceiling, inspecting the overhead tiles. He could hear Beltman arguing adamantly with the two officers outside the door. Hawthorn would've cried had he not been too exhausted to shed the tears. Geniomics had won. There was no way around it. He had nothing to combat their efforts.

Hawthorn picked up the phone and held it to his ear. Surprisingly, it still worked. He dialed Cindy's number and talked to a police sergeant who informed him that she was missing but that they had already initiated a search. Hawthorn's brow suddenly lightened. Apparently, they'd found a memo left on her answering machine. It was a message in Cindy's own voice. Three words: "Vonnegut's a champ." The pain seemed to quickly disappear. Hawthorn knew exactly what it meant.

VENGEANCE

CHAPTER FORTY-SIX

There's something exhilarating about cornering the market on a new drug. You provide humanity with something that can reduce their pain. You give them energy. Hope. Love. For a short while, you can be God. You can affect and direct their lives. Most importantly, though, you know you're going to make a killing.

These were the thoughts that circled through Edmonds' mind as he strode casually down the length of the auditorium's main aisle. In a matter of minutes, the world would know that his company would place the first ever cure for the common cold on the shelves of every neighborhood pharmacy. Geniomics' colors, captured in each blue and white capsule, would be consumed by almost every person across the globe. A press conference was already lined up with every major international news team present. It was to be held shortly after the announcement at an adjacent hotel in the most lavishly rented conference room in all of San Francisco.

Edmonds could see Dr. Williams enter the building and slowly make his way towards Geniomics' executive team, who occupied the second and third rows. Edmonds smiled. All of his big dogs were there: Crooks from Finance, Simon from R&D, even Heathcrow from PR.

"Where the hell is Camden?" Edmonds asked. Crooks shrugged his shoulders. Camden had flown separately from Seattle. He'd stayed at the same hotel, but had arranged for his own transportation to the convention center. "That stupid son-of-a-bitch better get here on time. The press wants to talk to him more than anyone. They die for marketing BS."

Crooks nodded his head and then shrugged his shoulders a second time.

"I'll fire his ass as soon the market settles."

Edmonds twisted in his seat and could see Williams stopping to shake hands with anyone related to the medical field. The plan had come together. Enjoy your handshakes, Allen, he thought. You nearly screwed the entire thing up. Edmonds shot a quick smile to an analyst sitting two rows back. He looked at Williams who paused nervously in the aisle. He was looking at someone seated towards the side of the auditorium. That's when Edmonds smile turned upside down.

Hawthorn was sitting boldly in a side aisle fifteen rows back with a woman holding him tightly by the hand. On one side was an Italian man who whispered quietly in Hawthorn's ear. Occasionally, Hawthorn would twist and talk to three people sitting in the row behind them.

*   *   *   *   *   *   *   *

Hawthorn could see Williams lean in close and whisper something into Edmonds' ear, his bony finger pointing in Hawthorn's direction. Unimpressed, Edmonds flashed Hawthorn a thin smile and then returned his attention to the stage. The lights flickered and everyone took their seats.

Seven members of the ICC's executive committee emerged from behind the stage to take their seats on the other side of a long walnut table. Draped across its edge was a green banner holding the seal of the International Conservation Consortium.

The commissioner general leaned forward, bringing the microphone close to his mouth. His voice was deep and commanding and sounded with a dignified English accent. "I'd like to welcome everyone to this hearing: each of you from industry, the medical fields, members of the press. I know you've all worked very hard to get to this point. Let me first begin by saying that the medical field is one that has evolved since the first human beings walked across the face of this earth. With this long tradition come some of the greatest discoveries in the history of mankind. Every day an individual in this industry takes one step closer to curing an ailment previously untreated."

Edmonds looked arrogantly forward as a flashcube sparkled from the side of the room. His mind was already working on his opening line and how he'd get the reporters fired up.

"Each time our researchers make a single positive step in these directions, they give this field the building blocks to move forward with greater determination. With greater purpose. So we proceed along this path as one discovery leads to another. And then another. To this degree, we have been given the power to create. The power to make things that previously did not exist. But we are not gods. These powers must be used in a delicate balance with the natural world in which we live."

Hawthorn shifted nervously in his seat.

"With each discovery comes the battle for market share, global dominance, and profits. As imperfect beings, we encounter the temptation to misuse these resources in the name of greed and wealth. This consortium committee sitting before you, made up of seven international members, was assembled to discourage that very lure: to protect our surroundings, the environment and our people. It is for this very reason that this group *denies* Geniomics approval for the use of the Conrava Goliath species."

The Geniomics team was in shock. Outraged, Edmonds rose to his feet. "What in the hell is going on here?"

The commissioner's voice boomed through the auditorium's speakers. "Denied, sir, because *we-will-not* condone the falsification of test results."

362

"Stop right-"

"Step down, sir. I am not finished."

Edmonds was furious. "How can you-"

"Denied, for misleading the global community, Mr. Edmonds."

"This is an outrage-"

"And denied, sir, for tampering with human lives. The approval hearing for R2-X is closed. This committee will reconvene two hours from now." The commissioner slammed the gavel to the small wooden pad as Edmonds pleaded his case to the exiting committee.

"Can somebody please tell me what in God's name is happening here?"

Flashes of lights from a battalion of reporters sparkled throughout the room.

"Do something!" Edmonds screamed to his legal team. Each of them stood paralyzed by the moment. He grabbed Williams and pulled him toward the side of the auditorium where a small flight of stairs would lead them backstage. "What the fuck is going on here? Explain this to me, Allen!"

Williams shook his head. He appeared as astonished as anyone. "We just have to talk to them, Randy. I'm sure it's a misunderstanding. A mix-up."

"I don't give- You get us back there, Allen. You're the one who's friends with these idiots."

The two men were met at the base of the stairs by a security guard refusing to allow them passage. While Williams argued, Edmonds looked over the crowd. Descending rapidly down one of the auditorium's aisles was a group of FDA officers. At the top of the stairs, he could see Dr. Hawthorn making his way to the door.

*   *   *   *   *   *   *   *

The first person Hawthorn thanked was Howard. Sensing he was in trouble earlier in the week, Mason had hidden one of his own vials inside Hawthorn's Slyvy-M refrigeration unit. Hawthorn had asked Cindy to record his numbers before his trip to Seattle. Running late, she was forced to take some vials home with her in a portable cooler. When she realized what she had in her possession, she called Howard and left the sample with him at the gate.

The next person he thanked was Ken Camden. Cindy's friends inside Geniomics had heard rumors that the VP of Marketing did not agree with the testing techniques and, after Hawthorn informed them that Cindy was missing, they decided to contact him. Camden easily agreed to cooperate and supply the ICC with detailed records of his meeting minutes as well as several bits of research data he knew had been fabricated.

Lastly was Dr. Clark, the only one with enough clout to move on Hawthorn's allegations. He quickly contacted Dan Schwartz to formulate a legal strategy to protect the Center as well as contact the ICC.

Surrounded by a mob of reporters and glimmering flashes of light, both Edmonds and Williams were escorted up the main aisle. As they passed, Edmonds stared at Hawthorn coldly and Williams smiled sarcastically from behind.

"I'll be in touch," Edmonds barked.

Hawthorn suddenly broke from Jordan's grasp, barging his way between the guards and shoving Edmonds aside. He drew back his fist and struck Williams square in the jaw. Hawthorn buckled over as his ribs cracked free again. The group of officers quickly pulled Hawthorn away as they lifted an angry Williams from the ground to move him through the door. "That's for your sister."

Jordan held him close as the group made their way out of the building. His ribs ached with pain and he desperately needed to sleep. Hawthorn still didn't know for sure who had killed Mason's patients and, for all intents and purposes, it was too late to find that out. Xiao had abruptly left the country and the authorities were in the process of trying to work a deal to get him back.

Hawthorn draped his arm around Jordan's shoulder and kissed her on the top of her head. It was a new beginning. A fresh start. After all, he was a doctor. And he had lives to save.

-2000-

Three years after Mason's tragic death, Hawthorn visited the Old County Library that Mason had described to him in great detail. By now, Hawthorn had earned a high-ranking position on the hospital staff as Dr. Clark rewarded him handsomely for his sacrifice.

The fall out from Hawthorn's effort was enormous. The Commissioner of the FDA had been asked to resign amid a full-scale, Congress-led investigation. The entire pharmaceutical industry and political circuit was now locked in debate around the role and ramifications of industry-funded political action councils in medicine.

Triton bestowed upon the CME a large financial donation for Hawthorn's help in exposing Geniomics' lie. With Edmonds behind bars, R2-X was now being redesigned at the CME by cutting-edge virotherapists who would employ the drug to locate the cold-causing adenovirus and then inject it with genetic instructions to target and destroy cancer cells. It was decided that part of the commercial proceeds would be shared with the millions of volunteers who had unknowingly donated compute time to R2-X's original research.

Cindy, as it turns out, had been found in a nearby hotel room bound and gagged. And although traumatic, she appeared to quickly recover and continue her research at the CME.

Jordan and Hawthorn eventually moved into a comfortable three-bedroom home with plenty of room for his new son to roam and play. They acquired two dogs and a cat named "Bearcloud" who had a knack for finding his way into bad situations. He also made a trip home to see his father, who weeks later fell to the debilitating disease.

Of course, Hawthorn and Jordan never again traveled back to the forest. Never once did they discuss it. It was something they wanted to forget, a memory to be buried with the past.

Hawthorn walked with his head cocked backwards, staring up at the high ceilings of the library. Everything he saw appeared exactly as Mason had said. He could almost hear Mason's voice commentating with each step he took.

After navigating through the large reference section, he found the aisles on the second level that cradled the older books. It was quiet up there. There were no librarians putting away books or visitors milling about. It was as if the air stood still. Mason was right. You could almost feel the ghosts rushing past you.

At eye level Hawthorn could see that the books in this section were dedicated to psychology. He compared the call numbers on the small piece of paper in his hand with those on the books. Hawthorn had found these numbers in Mason's apartment when the authorities were going through his things. The titles read: <u>Dementia</u>, <u>Criminal Psychology</u>, <u>West's Guide to Psychotic Disorders</u>, and <u>Multiple Personality Syndrome</u>. He reached out and withdrew a book entitled, <u>The Schizophrenic Mind</u>.

"A boring edition if you ask me," a man's voice said. Hawthorn jumped. There was no one there. "There are much better books than that."

The voice was coming from the other side of the shelves. Hawthorn removed a few texts and then reached through the shelves moving a couple more. It was Beltman. He'd been missing since the ICC hearing.

"What are you doing here?"

"Oh, I thought I'd do a little reading. You know, expand my mind." He held up a copy of the latest <u>American Journal of Psychology</u>. "Have you seen the lead article?"

"What article?" Hawthorn asked, peering through the small opening at Beltman's plastic hair.

"Quite fascinating, actually. A boy watches his mother kill his father and then spends the rest of his life trying to kill her even though she's already dead." Beltman mused over his own words. "How touching. Funny how Mason was able to forget all that... at least for a little while.

"How do you-"

"How do you think, John? Humm?" A wry smile traveled from ear to ear. Beltman glanced at his watch, an expensive Bavarian model. On the top of his left hand was the scar from a very deep wound. "My it's getting late."

He took the journal and placed it carefully under a stack of three books. "There we go. Now it's buried."

Hawthorn felt like slamming the entire shelf down upon him.

"Oh, don't get so upset, Hawthorn," Beltman said, looking over the stacks of books. "After all, a library's sort of a graveyard, isn't it?"

THE END.